T0296398

Intraoperative Ultrasound (IOUS) in Neurosurgery

Francesco Prada • Luigi Solbiati
Alberto Martegani • Francesco DiMeco
Editors

Intraoperative Ultrasound (IOUS) in Neurosurgery

From Standard B-mode to Elastosonography

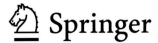

Editors

Francesco Prada
Istituto Neurologico C. Besta
Fondazione IRCCS
Milano
Italy

Alberto Martegani
UO Radiologia
Ospedale Valduce
Como
Italy

Luigi Solbiati
UO Radiologia Oncologica
Humanitas Univ. and Research Hospital
Busto Arsizio
Italy

Francesco DiMeco
Istituto Neurologico C. Besta
Fondazione IRCCS
Milano
Italy

ISBN 978-3-319-25266-7   ISBN 978-3-319-25268-1   (eBook)
DOI 10.1007/978-3-319-25268-1

Library of Congress Control Number: 2016931308

Springer Cham Heidelberg New York Dordrecht London

Printed on acid-free paper

Springer International Publishing AG Switzerland is part of Springer Science+Business Media (www.springer.com)

Preface

Seeing is believing: intraoperative imaging has always been of great help in finding and defining different brain and spinal lesions, and neurosurgeons have always had a great interest in its development. Many tools are available: neuronavigation has been for years a standard tool in almost every neurosurgical unit, but it has the limitations of being based on preoperative imaging which cannot be updated.

Intraoperative computed tomography (iCT) and magnetic resonance imaging (iMRI) have become a standard intraoperative tool, despite not being true real-time tools that can provide direct guidance, and being costly and time consuming; however, image interpretation is straightforward.

This is probably related to the fact that CT and MRI are the main diagnostic tool for CNS pathologies and all neurosurgeons are accustomed to it.

This is not the case of ultrasounds (US), which are scarcely used for adult cerebral and spinal diagnostics, except for some vascular diseases, and therefore represent a sort of "gray area" for neurosurgeons, neuroradiologists, and radiologists and for even those interested in ultrasound.

iUS has been used in neurosurgery since the 1960s, with the pioneering work of Dyck et al., and are still under development. Despite becoming more widespread, they still are far from being considered a routine tool and fully understood in their great potential by the neurosurgical community.

Some authors, prior to this work, tried to standardize this technique and define basic rules to apply into the neurosurgical theater, as it is the case for other parts of the human body. It has to be noted that it is difficult to transmit to the reader the multiple features and opportunities offered by US application in neurosurgery: images are usually taken from examinations that last for some minutes and represents only partially the findings. Videos obtained during the examination are by far more complete and contribute to the understanding of the underlying anatomy, but do not include the manual movement of the US probe that allows the surgeon to translate the two-dimensional US findings into the three-dimensional surgical field within the brain, spinal cord, and nerves. US is also an operator-dependant technique, and the ability to set different parameters is pivotal to obtain good quality imaging. Therefore the machine commands have also to be understood by the surgeon, which add further difficulties to an already complex task. In fact the intraoperative setting differs completely from its diagnostic counterpart and rules apply differently. Furthermore in the past, due to technical limitations, US imaging was very poor, especially compared to CT and MRI, and this also did not contribute to its use as a surgical tool. Moreover, the lack of standardization, specific knowledge, and training contribute to the consideration of iUS as an adjunct rather than a stand-alone tool in the neurosurgical armamentarium.

In the last years, there have been major technical advances which benefitted greatly the quality of US images that are now comparable in terms of spatial resolution and are by far superior in terms of temporal resolution and readiness to those obtained with iCT or iMRI.

The intraoperative use of US has been refined and made more understandable, for example, with the use of high-resolution power Doppler and 3D navigation, and interesting additional features, such as the use of ultrasound contrast agents or elastosonography, are under investigation.

Our aim of this book is to bring to the attention of the neurosurgical and radiological community the recent advances in sonology and their great potential for the application of intraoperative ultrasound in neurosurgery, relying on the experience gathered by leading experts in different fields.

We will address all the advantages and disadvantages of this great real-time intraoperative tool, always keeping in mind that the full exploitation is achievable through a synergistic effort between neurosurgeons, neuroradiologists, and sonologists, bringing together all different clinical needs.

Therefore, in the first part of the book, we addressed and explained the physics and basic principles of ultrasound, as well as its major clinical application.

We then explore the use of standard B-mode and Doppler, from the semeiotics to exam execution and machine setting in general radiology, and then we tried to translate this experience in the field of neurosurgery aiming at a standardization of the US experience: machine settings for brain, spine, and peripheral nerves evaluation, how to perform the examination, major anatomical topographical and pathological US findings.

In the following chapters, advanced US techniques such as fusion imaging for virtual navigation, contrast-enhanced ultrasound, and elastosonography are highlighted, discussing their application in already standardized body districts, such as the liver, and their application, potential role, and future exploitation in neurosurgery.

We truly believe that IOUS will progressively become a pivotal tool for intraoperative imaging in neurosurgery and that its multiple features and future development will lead to new frontiers in intraoperative imaging and therapeutics, such as the possibility to detect tumor remnants with CEUS or elastosonosgraphy, deliver chemotherapeutic agents using microbubbles, control tumor regrowth, or deliver high-focused ultrasound through artificial ultrasound compatible bone flap. We hope that this book will provide some explanations and answers to the most common questions in this regard, but also highlight the multiple possibilities still to be exploited.

Milano, Italy   Francesco Prada
Busto Arsizio, Italy   Luigi Solbiati
Como, Italy   Alberto Martegani
Milano, Italy   Francesco DiMeco

Acknowledgments

I wish to thank Dr. Francesco DiMeco, my "Chief", for having recognized the value and potential of IOUS, and for continuously pushing towards improvement, and my mentor, Dr. Sergio Giombini, who encouraged the use of IOUS despite his diffidence towards new technologies. I am also indebted to Dr. Gigi Solbiati and Dr. Alberto Martegani, cutting-edge radiologists, who became interested in the application of US in neurosurgery, recognized its potential, and patiently shared their knowledge in the field during many discussions.

Credit should also be given to Luca Lodigiani, colleague and friend, who shared this obsession and endangered his job in order to pursue this project.

I would also like to thank my parents, particularly my father, recognized clinician, who kept on telling me to write clinical experiences. I hope this is enough.

A special thank you to Caroline and Antonia, my wife and daughter, who tolerate my absence, both physical and mental, and continuously support me in my endeavor to meet the demands of a job as challenging as neurosurgery, allowing me to have a "normal" life.

Francesco Prada, MD

About the Editors

Dr. Francesco Prada is staff neurosurgeon in the 1st Neurosurgical Division of the Department of Neurosurgery at the Fondazione IRCCS Istituto Neurologico C.Besta in Milan, Italy, where he received his surgical training with Professor S. Giombini, before starting to cooperate with Professor F. DiMeco.

Dr. Prada shares his interest between clinical practice and research, with main interest in skull base surgery and neuro-oncology.

He is currently leading the "Intra-operative Ultrasound in Neurosurgery Project", started in 2009, and has in fact performed more than 500 image-guided ultrasound procedures.

He particularly focuses on the intraoperative applications of ultrasound for the treatment of cerebral and spinal tumor and vascular lesions. He is currently developing advanced ultrasound techniques in neurosurgery, such as fusion Imaging for virtual navigation, contrast-enhanced ultrasound (CEUS), and elastosonography.

His interest for diagnostic and therapeutic US applications lead to his involvement in the "TheraGlio" project, aimed at the development of multimodal contrast agents.

He has further interest in alpinism and has obtained the diploma in mountain medicine of the "Union Internationale des Associations d'Alpinisme"; he is currently investigating the physiopathological mechanism of cerebral edema in high altitude mountain sickness.

Dr. Prada has published numerous original articles in peer-reviewed journals and chapters in textbooks of *Neurosurgery* and has been editor and reviewer of numerous scientific publications. He has given presentations and lectures at national and international meetings.

Luigi Solbiati was Chairman of the Department of Oncology and Head of the Division of Interventional Oncologic Radiology at the Hospital of Busto Arsizio (Milan, Italy) for 13 years and has been Contract Professor of Techniques and Methods of Diagnostic Imaging at the University of Milan since 1988. In July 2015, he became Professor of Radiology at Humanitas University and Research Hospital in Milan. His main fields of interest have always been small parts ultrasound, interventional procedures in oncologic diseases (particularly tumor ablation), imaging of the neck, and contrast-enhanced sonography. He was one of the pioneers of ultrasound-guided aspiration biopsies (1979), ethanol injection of solid tumors (1983), and fusion imaging for the guidance of interventional procedures (2003). He has one of the largest world experiences in the treatment of liver malignancies with radiofrequency ablation (RFA) and, more recently, high-power microwaves, accounting for more than 2200 patients. Prof. Solbiati has published 112 original articles in peer-reviewed journals and 81 chapters in textbooks of Radiology, Interventional Radiology, and Oncology and has been editor of 11 books on small parts sonography, contrast-enhanced sonography, and ablative therapies. He has given more than 550 presentations at Meetings in 36 different countries. In 2006, Prof. Solbiati chaired the first World Conference on Interventional Oncology (Cernobbio, Italy) and in 2013 the first Interventional Oncology Sans Frontieres Congress (IOSFC) (Cernobbio, Italy). His H-index is currently 41, his impact factor exceeds 400, and his publications had more than 10,800 citations.

Dr. Alberto Martegani is Director of the Department of Radiology of the Valduce Hospital, Como. He started his career as a radiologist in 1981 under the guidance of Prof. Carlo Del Favero and Prof. Mario Bianchi, covering all aspects of the radiological fields, mainly focusing his efforts towards interventional neuroradiology. He then shifted his education towards musculoskeletal radiology, while, in the early 1980s began to work with ultrasound. His subject of interests became abdominal diagnostics, along with the study of continuous wave Doppler and Duplex technology. In the same period, he applied the use of ultrasound for the intraoperative localization of brain lesions, in a first fruitful cooperation within the field of neurosurgery. Further interventional procedures were *percutaneous* discectomy, embolization, and angioplasty of the peripheral *arterial* system.

In the 1990s, he followed his "maestro", Dott. Carlo Del Favero, in Como, where he became Director in 2006, becoming not only a cutting-edge clinician but also a key developer for industries.

He pioneered the studies aimed at the development of algorithms for contrast-enhanced ultrasound and its possible clinical applications, along with the first clinical experiences on real-time elastosonography and fusion imaging for real-time ultrasound-based navigation. He also participated in studies on tissutal characterization with ultrasound radiofrequency.

Since he became Director of the Department of Radiology, he also started to study socio-sanitary issues such as cost-effectiveness in the field of ultrasound.

Dr. Martegani has published numerous articles in peer-reviewed journals along with chapters in textbooks and is editor and reviewer of numerous scientific publications. He has given presentations and lectures at national and international meetings and leads theoretical-practical courses on Doppler imaging.

Francesco DiMeco, MD, achieved his medical degree *summa cum laude* at the University of Milan in 1988 and completed his neurosurgical residency in 1993 at the same University. Then, he attended a neurosurgical oncology fellowship at Johns Hopkins University from 1997 to 2000. He is currently Director of the Department of Neurosurgery and Director of the Neurosurgical

Oncology Division at the Fondazione Istituto Neurologico C.Besta of Milan. He is also appointed as Assistant Professor (adjunct), within the Department of Neurological Surgery at Johns Hopkins Medical School and as part-time Professor of Neurosurgery at the University of Milan. He is mainly interested in brain tumors and skull base surgery. His research areas of interest include identifying and testing novel antitumor agents, including anti-angiogenic factors locally delivered by polymers; combined use of different classes of anti-cancer drugs; use of genetically engineered stem cells to locally deliver antitumor agents for brain tumors; brain tumor stem cells; and intraoperative imaging for image guided resection of brain tumors. He is the coordinator of the Theraglio Project within the 7th Framework Program of the European Community. Francesco DiMeco has published several scientific articles in Medline indexed journals, among which four reviews and nine book chapters. He is also coeditor of a scientific textbook. He serves as ad hoc reviewer for several scientific journals and member of the editorial board of Journal of Neuro-Oncology.

Contents

Contributors

Luca Aiani Department of Radiology, Ospedale Valduce, Como, Italy

Jeffrey Bamber Joint Department of Physics, Institute of Cancer Research and The Royal Marsden Hospital, Sutton, UK

Valentina Caldiera, MD Neuroradiology Unit, Fondazione IRCCS Istituto Neurologico C. Besta, Milan, Italy

Luigi Caputi, MD Department of Cerebrovascular Diseases, Fondazione IRCCS Istituto Neurologico C. Besta, Milan, Italy

Daniela Caremani Department of Infectious Diseases, Section of Anatomical Pathology, Ospedale S. Donato, Arezzo, Italy

Marcello Caremani, MD Radiology Unit, Department of Infectious Diseases, Ospedale S. Donato, Arezzo, Italy

Aabir Chakraborty Wessex Neurological Centre, Southampton General Hospital, Southampton, UK

Huan Wee Chan Victor Horsley Department of Neurosurgery, The National Hospital for Neurology and Neurosurgery, London, UK

Elisa Ciceri, MD Neuroradiology Unit, Fondazione IRCCS Istituto Neurologico C. Besta, Milan, Italy

Jan Coburger Department of Neurosurgery, University of Ulm, Günzburg, Germany

Massimiliano Del Bene, MD Department of Neurosurgery, Fondazione IRCCS Istituto Neurologico C. Besta, Milan, Italy

Francesco DiMeco Department of Neurosurgery, Fondazione IRCCS Istituto Neurologico C. Besta, Milan, Italy

Department of Neurological Surgery, Johns Hopkins Medical School, Baltimore, MD, USA

Neil Dorward Victor Horsley Department of Neurosurgery, The National Hospital for Neurology and Neurosurgery, London, UK

Carlo Giussani Department of Neurosurgery, University of Milano-Bicocca, San Gerardo University Hospital, Monza, Italy

Ralph W. König Department of Neurosurgery, University of Ulm, Günzburg, Germany

Alberto Martegani, MD Department of Radiology, Ospedale Valduce, Como, Italy

Luca Mattei Department of Neurosurgery, Fondazione IRCCS Istituto Neurologico C. Besta, Milan, Italy

Giovanni Mauri, MD Department of Radiology, Policlinico San Donato, San Donato Milanese (Milano), Italy

Department of Interventional Radiology, European Institute of Oncology, Milano, Italy

Alessandro Moiraghi Department of Neurosurgery, Fondazione IRCCS Istituto Neurologico C. Besta, Milan, Italy

Aliasgar V. Moiyadi, MCh Neurosurgery Services, Department of Surgical Oncology, Tata Memorial Centre and Advanced Centre for Treatment Research and Education in Cancer (ACTREC), Parel, Mumbai, India

Maria Teresa Pedro Department of Neurosurgery, University of Ulm, Günzburg, Germany

Francesco Prada, MD Department of Neurosurgery, Fondazione IRCCS Istituto Neurologico C. Besta, Milan, Italy

Carla Richetta Department of Neurosurgery, Fondazione IRCCS Istituto Neurologico C. Besta, Milan, Italy

Matteo Riva Department of Neurosurgery, University of Milano-Bicocca, San Gerardo University Hospital, Monza, Italy

Luca Maria Sconfienza, MD, PhD Institute of Radiology, Università degli Studi di Milano, San Donato Milanese, Italy

Radiology Unit, IRCCS Policlinico San Donato, San Donato Milanese, Italy

Francesco Secchi, MD Department of Biomedical Sciences for Health, Università degli Studi di Milano, Milan, Italy

Prakash Shetty, MCh Neurosurgery Services, Department of Surgical Oncology, Tata Memorial Centre and Advanced Centre for Treatment Research and Education in Cancer (ACTREC), Parel, Mumbai, India

Luigi Solbiati Department of Biomedical Sciences, Humanitas University Department of Radiology, Humanitas Research Hospital Rozzano (Milano), Italy

Andrej Šteňo, MD, PhD Department of Neurosurgery, Comenius University Faculty of Medicine, University Hospital Bratislava, Bratislava, Slovakia

Christopher Uff Victor Horsley Department of Neurosurgery, The National Hospital for Neurology and Neurosurgery, London, UK

Geirmund Unsgård, MD, PhD Neurosurgical Department, St Olav University Hospital and Norwegian University of Science and Technology, Trondheim, Norway

Ignazio G. Vetrano, MD Department of Neurosurgery, Fondazione IRCCS Istituto Neurologico C. Besta, Milan, Italy

Università degli Studi di Milano, Milan, Italy

Part I

General Aspects

Clinical Ultrasound: Historical Aspects

1

Prakash Shetty and Aliasgar V. Moiyadi

Ultrasound has been used in medical imaging for over six decades. It is one of the most widely used technologies for diagnostic as well as therapeutic purposes. Ultrasound is popular compared to other diagnostic modalities because it is non-radioactive, portable and relatively cheap. Technically, ultrasound waves are sound waves having frequency above the threshold for human hearing (20 kHz).

1.1 Origins of Ultrasound Imaging

The history of ultrasound dates back to the mid-1700s with the postulation of the existence of non-audible sounds (Lazzaro), the discovery of the piezoelectric effect and the Doppler phenomenon in the 1800s and the development of A-mode (1950s) and later B-mode dynamic scans (late 1970s) to present-day cutting-edge technology developing at a rapid pace [1].

Lazzaro Spallanzani (1729–1799), who was an Italian priest and physiologist, first proved the existence of non-audible sound. In a series of detailed experiments on bats, he found that they could fly without colliding into obstacles in total darkness. He hypothesised that bats navigated using sound waves rather than sight in darkness (echolocation). Johann Christian Doppler (1803–1853) was an Austrian physicist who put forward a hypothesis stating that the observed frequency of a wave depends on the relative speed of the source and the observer. According to this effect (subsequently called the Doppler effect), if the source was moving towards the observer, then the observed frequency of the wave would be higher, and when moving away from the observer, it was lower. Today, this effect is routinely used to determine the velocity and direction of blood flow and helps in the imaging of blood vessels using ultrasound. In 1880, the French physicist Pierre Curie and his brother Jacques Curie discovered the piezoelectric phenomenon in some solids. The piezoelectric effect stated that some solids like quartz when subjected to mechanical stress generated electrical charge, and further, the reverse phenomenon was also possible. This important principle was used later to develop ultrasound transducers which produced ultrasonic waves on application of electric current and were able to reconvert the reflected sound waves into electrical signals for generation of an ultrasound image. As with other technologies, further advances in ultra-

P. Shetty, MCh • A.V. Moiyadi, MCh (✉)
Neurosurgery Services, Department of Surgical Oncology, Tata Memorial Centre and Advanced Centre for Treatment Research and Education in Cancer (ACTREC),
1221, HBB, Tata Memorial Hospital E Borges Road, Parel, Mumbai 400012, India
e-mail: aliasgar.moiyadi@gmail.com

© Springer International Publishing Switzerland 2016
F. Prada et al. (eds.), *Intraoperative Ultrasound (IOUS) in Neurosurgery: From Standard B-mode to Elastosonography*, DOI 10.1007/978-3-319-25268-1_1

sound owed its development to war. The French government called upon Paul Langevin, one of the Curie brothers' first students, to develop a device capable of detecting enemy submarines in the First World War. He along with a Russian immigrant engineer, Constantin Chilowsky, built such a device based on ultrasound technology in 1915. Reginald Aubrey Fessenden (1866–1932) built the first working SONAR system for echolocation using the principle of detecting reflected sound waves in 1914. It could detect icebergs in sea up to 2 miles away. In 1928, Soviet physicist Sergei Sokolov suggested the use of ultrasound technology for detecting flaws in metal sheets and joints.

1.2 Intraoperative Ultrasound and Neurosurgery

The use of ultrasound in medicine was a result of ingenious individuals trying to adapt ultrasound technology, which was already in use by the military and maritime industry. The initial ultrasound images were graphical representations in the form of A-mode scan and later on developed into recognisable anatomical patterns as seen in the B-mode scan imaging. Karl Theodore Dussik was a pioneer in using ultrasound for brain imagining and is called the father of ultrasonic diagnosis. He was a neurologist from the University of Vienna and as early as 1941, presented his idea of using ultrasound as a diagnostic tool. The first ultrasound images of the brain and ventricles, obtained with the help of an early prototype built by Dussik and his brother Friedrich, were published in 1947. They called the procedure "hyperphonography". This was the first attempt at imaging a human organ. They used a through-transmission technique with two transducers on either side of the head to produce the image. Later in 1952, it emerged that the images presumed to be of the ventricle were in fact a result of the artefact of the skull bone, and the transmission technique was abandoned in favour of reflection technique which was subsequently used by all pioneering centres in Europe, the United States and Japan.

1.2.1 A-Mode Scan Period

A (amplitude modulation)-mode scan ultrasound was the earliest single dimensional graphical ultrasound imaging method. A single transducer was used to produce as well as collect the reflected ultrasound. The X-axis represented the distance of the object from the transducer and the Y-axis represented the amplitude of the reflected wave (echo). Echogenic objects were characterised on the basis of amplitude and the time of occurrence of the wave on the ultrasound plot. This type of scan is still used in modern ophthalmology where measurements of various chambers are more important than anatomical details (Fig. 1.1). The use of A-mode ultrasound for localisation of brain tumour was investigated by French et al. (1950), using post-mortem specimens of cerebral

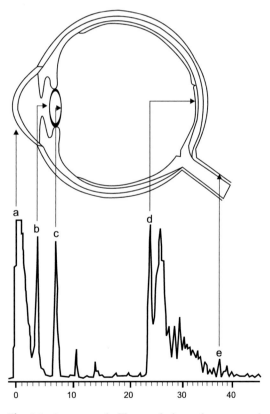

Fig. 1.1 A-scan graph: The *graph* shows the waves and their amplitude reflected off various structures of the eye, viz., (**a**) anterior surface of the cornea, (**b**) anterior surface of the lens, (**c**) posterior surface of the lens, (**d**) retina and (**e**) retroglobe structures

neoplasms, which showed increased reflectivity as compared to the normal brain [2]. William Peyton, a neurosurgeon, was the first to use ultrasound in an operating theatre for tumour localisation in a patient suffering from parietal glioblastoma in 1951 [3]. The tumour also showed an increased echogenic pattern as seen in the previous post-mortem studies. There were many reports by various authors looking into the possible use of echoencephalography in brain tumour surgery [4–6]. Tanaka et al. (1965) were able to image tumours in the frontal and temporal lobes preoperatively through the intact skull using a 2.25 MHz transducer using the reflection technique and confirmed them intraoperatively or during autopsy [7]. Walker and Uematsu tried to characterise various brain lesion intraoperatively using a 5 mHz formalin sterilised probe [8]. They found that the acoustic characteristic in case of low-grade astrocytoma was similar to the normal brain, and it was difficult to differentiate the margins of the tumour. Other high-grade tumours, cysts, metastases and meningiomas produced identifiable acoustic patterns. Backlund (1975) used the ultrasound along with the stereotactic Leksell frame to identify various echo-producing structures in the biopsy path [9]. The A-scan obtained from the planned biopsy path was overlaid on the stereotactic films of the patient to identify various solid and cystic structures based on the A-scan echo data. Several other authors described the intraoperative imaging properties of various tumours. There was also an attempt at correlating the ultrasound wave pattern with the tumour histology. This did not yield any conclusive results, but the role of ultrasound in tumour localisation during surgery was established.

1.2.2   The B-Scan Period

The B-mode ultrasound was devised in the late 1940s and was available for commercial use in the early 1960s. It was less popular than A-mode ultrasound till the late 1970s as it was bulky, difficult to use and had poor depth penetration. B-mode ultrasound is a two-dimensional imaging method obtained by moving the transducer in a plane above the object. The image obtained was the tomogram (slice view) of the object. The magnitude of reflected echo is displayed as brightness of a point (hence, the name B = "brightness" mode). The first B-mode images were simple black or white pictures. However, the use of grey-scale imaging was a critical step in generating vivid, easily identifiable anatomical images (Fig. 1.2) and increasing the popularity of ultrasound [10].

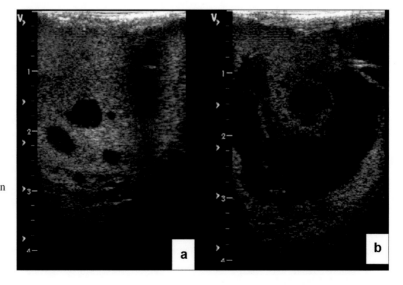

Fig. 1.2 (**a**, **b**) Typical B-scan dynamic mode imaging pictures of an intracranial glioma showing heterogeneous (mixed hyperechoic and anechoic areas) mass

Meanwhile in the late 1970s and early 1980s, the CT and MRI imaging technology provided imaging which had resolution not seen until then, with highly accurate details about tumour location and dimension. This prompted more neurosurgical procedures as more lesions were detected. There was a need for safe intraoperative method for localising the subcortical lesion to minimise damage, which the CT and MRI failed to provide. The development of 2D real-time sector scanning ultrasound revolutionised the use of ultrasonography in the intraoperative setting. Rubin in 1980 published a preliminary report of real-time ultrasound scanning using a rotating sector scanner in two cases of brain tumours and emphasised the role of ultrasound in visualising brain structures during surgery [11]. Rubin along with Dohrmann developed probes with three different frequencies for neurosurgical use – 3, 5 and 7.5 MHz. Simultaneously, others also published their observation about real-time ultrasound scanning in brain surgeries [12, 13]. Masuzawa published 54 cases of intraoperative sector scanning and found that ultrasound was 89 % helpful in 19 cases of supratentorial lesion, with no cortical injury or infections [14]. Koivukangas reported the first European study on real-time sector scanning during brain surgery and emphasised the importance of ultrasound in defining pathological anatomy [15]. Chandler et al. using real-time sector scanner in 18 cases of tumour surgery stressed on the critical assistance in localisation of subcortical tumour by ultrasound [16]. There were many difficulties and pitfalls earlier, described by Pasto (1984), especially in case of low-grade gliomas whose image characteristic closely resembles the normal brain. It required experience to detect the subtle mass effect due to the tumour in such cases [17]. The use of ultrasound intraoperatively increased during the 1980s, with new applications being reported. Shkolnik (1981) reported the use of intraoperative ultrasonography for placement of ventriculo-peritoneal shunt tube in infants with hydrocephalus and also for cystoperitoneal shunt for an infant with midline brain cyst [18]. Enzmann (1984) reported the use of intraoperative ultrasonography through a burr hole using a small 5 mHz transducer in five patients. The images obtained closely matched the computed tomographic images and helped in performing brain biopsies in these patients [19]. Berger et al. in 1986 developed an ultrasound-based stereotactic device that permitted biopsies of intracranial lesion through a burr hole, with visualisation of pre-, intra- and post-procedure status of the lesion using ultrasound [20]. Compared with CT-based stereotactic frames, the procedure time was less and complications like hematoma could be detected early after the biopsy. It was also useful in paediatric patients as the need for general anaesthesia during transport to the CT scanner was also avoided. Over the years, CT- and MRI-based frame and frameless systems have gained popularity for localisation and biopsy. However, still many centres prefer the ultrasound as a handy tool for biopsy. Also, if there is an error during calculation or if the stereotactic frame becomes loose, then the ultrasound becomes an important adjunct for biopsy. Development of portable ultrasound scanners has facilitated the use of US conveniently during neurosurgical procedures (Fig. 1.3).

1.3 Beyond 2D US

The 2D ultrasound continued to be used throughout the 1980s and 1990s. One of the drawbacks with the 2D ultrasound was the problem with orientation and the need to continuously see the instrument in the field while navigating. Koivukangas described an ultrasound holographic B (UHB) imaging technique [21]. This was a very early attempt at reconstructing 2D US data. It essentially utilised not only the amplitude of the reflected echo but also the phase which could accurately depict the position of the particular echo. Despite its early promise, UHB imaging did not gain much clinical application. Since then, the development of navigation and 3D ultrasound technology in the last decade has solved many of the issues plaguing conventional B-mode imaging (Fig. 1.4). Navigated US has emerged as a very useful and reliable tool for resection control.

From the early days of limited A-scan US to the present era of high-resolution navigated 3D ultrasound images, US technology has evolved in leaps and bounds, empowering the neurosurgeon and supplementing the therapeutic armamentarium at the neurosurgeon's disposal.

Fig. 1.3 A portable modern
ultrasound scanner for intraoperative
use (SonoSite M-turbo; SonoSite Inc,
Bothell, WA, USA)

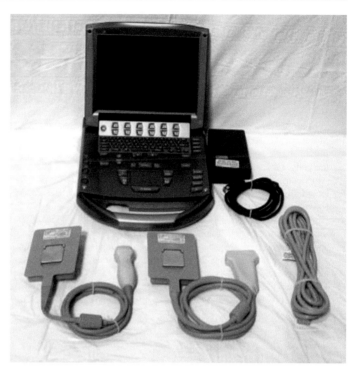

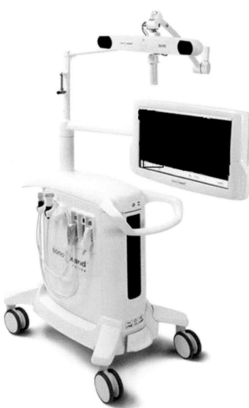

Fig. 1.4 A 3D ultrasound-based intraoperative imaging
and navigation system (SonoWand Invite™. SONOWAND
AS, Trondheim, Norway)

References

1. Newman PG, Rozycki GS (1998) The history of ultrasound. Surg Clin North Am 78(2):179–195
2. French LA, Wild JJ, Neal D (1950) Detection of cerebral tumors by ultrasonic pulses; pilot studies on postmortem material. Cancer 3(4):705–708
3. Wild JJ, Reid JM (1953) The effects on biological tissue of 15-mc pulsed ultrasound. J Acoust Soc Am 25:270–280
4. Tanaka K, Kikuchi Y, Uchida R (1953) Ultrasonic diagnosis of intracranial disease. Proc Surg Soc Japan 53:242–243
5. Kikuchi Y, Uchida R, Tanaka K, Wagai T (1957) Early cancer diagnosis through ultrasonics. J Acoust Soc Am 29:824–833
6. Dyck P, Kurze T, Barrows HS (1966) Intraoperative ultrasonic encephalography of cerebral mass lesions. Bull Los Angeles Neurol Soc 31(3):114–124
7. Tanaka K, Ito K, Wagai T (1965) The localization of brain tumors by ultrasonic techniques. A clinical review of 111 cases. J Neurosurg 23(2):135–147
8. Walker AE, Euemasu S (1966) Dural echoencephalography. J Neurosurg 25(6):634–637
9. Backlund EO, Levander B, Greitz T (1975) Stereotactic exploration of brain tumours by ultrasound. Acta Radiol Diagn (Stockh) 16(2):117–122
10. Kossoff G, Garrett WJ (1972) Ultrasonic film echoscopy for placental localization. Aust N Z J Obstet Gynaecol 12(2):117–121
11. Rubin JM, Mirfakhraee M, Duda EE, Dohrmann GJ, Brown F (1980) Intraoperative ultrasound examination of the brain. Radiology 137(3):831–832

12. Voorhies RM, Patterson RH (1980) Prelimnary experience with intra-operative ultrasonographic localization of brain tumors. Radiol Nucl Med Mag 10:8–9
13. Masuzawa H, Hachiya J, Kamitami H, Sakai F, Sato J (1981) Intra-operative use of ultrasonography in neurosurgery. Abstract: seventh international congress of neurological surgery, Munchen, July 12–18, 1981. Published in Neurological Surgery, Supplement to Neurochirurgica
14. Masuzawa H, Kamitami H, Sato J, Sano K (1982) Intraoperative sector – scanning ultrasonography of the brain. Presented at the 51st annual meeting of the American association of neurological surgeons, Honolulu, 25–29 Apr 1982
15. Koivukangas J, Alasaarela E, Nystrom SH (1982) Ultrasound holographic (UHB) and intra-operative sector scanning of the human brain. Abstract. 34th annual meeting of the scandinavian neurosurgical society, Trondheim, June 16–19. Printed in Acta Neurochir 66 (3–4):248
16. Chandler WF, Knake JE, Gillicuddy JE, Lillehei KO, Silver TM (1982) Intraoperative use of real-time ultrasonography in neurosurgery. J Neurosurg 57(2):157–163
17. Pasto ME, Rifkin MD (1984) Intraoperative ultrasound examination of the brain: possible pitfalls in diagnosis and biopsy guidance. J Ultrasound Med 3(6):245–249
18. Shkolnik A, McLone DG (1981) Intraoperative real-time ultrasonic guidance of ventricular shunt placement in infants. Radiology 141(2):515–517
19. Enzmann DR, Irwin KM, Marshall WH, Silverberg GD, Britt RH, Hanbery JW (1984) Intraoperative sonography through a burr hole: guide for brain biopsy. AJNR Am J Neuroradiol 5(3):243–246
20. Berger MS (1986) Ultrasound-guided stereotaxic biopsy using a new apparatus. J Neurosurg 65(4):550–554
21. Koivukangas J, Alasaarela E,Nystrom SHM (1982) Ultrasound holographic (UHB) and intra-operative sector scanning of the human brain. Abstract: 34th annual meeting of the scandinavian neurosurgical society, Trondheim, June 16–19, 1982. Printed in Acta Neurochir 66(3–4):248

US Physics, Basic Principles, and Clinical Application

2

Alberto Martegani, Luca Mattei, and Luca Aiani

2.1 Introduction

Ultrasonography is an imaging method which is widely used in medicine and is based on the processing of the echo signal generated by the interaction between the matter and an ultrasound beam.

The application of ultrasound in medicine was developed starting from the primitive A-mode and B-mode static systems, borrowed from metallurgy and from military technologies, and exponentially implemented over the past decades with the realization of equipment presenting many interesting features. Among these are the capability of producing real-time images rendered in the gray scale and the possibility of making functional and morphological examinations of the blood flow phenomena with color and power Doppler analysis; of providing 3D volume analysis, in real time; and recently, of assessing tissue elasticity with elastographic systems and taking advantage of the capabilities of analysis of the microcirculation and organ damage due to

contrast media and algorithms dedicated to their analysis. The few notations below are not certainly meant to examine exhaustively the complex topic of physics of ultrasound but rather to be an essential explanatory hint and a stimulus to increase the physical basis underlying this fascinating world of images.

2.2 The Nature of Ultrasound

Sound is a modality of transmission of energy, in this case, mechanical energy that, similarly to the waves of the sea, takes place without energy conveyance but by means of transmission of the vibration of a particle of matter to a contiguous particle. For this reason, sound cannot be transmitted through a vacuum but must necessarily be provided with a physical medium to be able to propagate. From a physical point of view, sound can be described as a wave phenomenon, the sound wave, which can be defined according to the properties of typical wave phenomena: wavelength (λ), frequency (f) (which are related to each other by the equation $\lambda = 1/f$), amplitude which expresses the amount of energy transported and propagation speed which depends on the nature and temperature of the medium in which the sound propagates [1, 2].

Its units are meter for the wavelength; Hertz (Hz) for the frequency; watts/cm^2, Pascal (Pa),

A. Martegani, MD (✉) • L. Aiani
Department of Radiology, Ospedale Valduce,
Via Dante Alighieri 11, Como 22100, Italy
e-mail: radiologia@valduce.it

L. Mattei
Department of Neurosurgery, Fondazione
IRCCS Istituto Neurologico C. Besta, Milan, Italy

© Springer International Publishing Switzerland 2016
F. Prada et al. (eds.), *Intraoperative Ultrasound (IOUS) in Neurosurgery:
From Standard B-mode to Elastosonography*, DOI 10.1007/978-3-319-25268-1_2

or decibel (dB) for the width; and meter per second (m/s) for the speed of propagation. Ultrasound is a peculiar type of sound waves with very high frequencies (>20,000 Hz). Ultrasound systems applied to medicine make use of ultrasounds with a frequency of between 2×10 Hz and $18–20 \times 10^6$ Hz, that is, between 2 and 18–20 MHz with very short wavelengths and therefore with features that allow the study of the anatomical structures with a high spatial resolution. In fact, the theoretical axial spatial resolution depends on the equation $\lambda/2$, and it is therefore understood why high frequencies allow to obtain higher spatial resolution. Wavelength and thus its reciprocal, frequency, are together with the medium of propagation the determining elements of an important property of ultrasound, the ability of propagation, which is the distance to which ultrasound can be transmitted in the medium. This capability is related to the ratio 1 dB/cm/MHz from which derives that the higher is the frequency of ultrasound, the lower is the transmission capability in depth.

2.3 The Nature of the Medium in Which the Ultrasound Propagates

As described above, the nature of the medium in which ultrasound propagates affects the speed and capability of propagation. In particular, propagation velocity is directly proportional to the density of the medium (ρ, expressed in g/cm^3) and inversely proportional to its elasticity (i.e., the ability to regain its original shape after deformation). The set of the physical properties of the medium in the interaction with an ultrasonic beam is defined acoustic impedance (Z) that expresses the characteristics of the medium when opposing to the passage of the acoustic wave; its unit is Rayl (by the English scientist Rayleigh) [3].

The equation which expresses acoustic impedance is

$$Z = \rho \times c$$

Z (acoustic impedance)
ρ (density of the medium)
c (speed of sound in the medium)

2.4 Interaction between Ultrasound and Matter

The attenuation that the ultrasound beam undergoes when crossing a tissue, which is expressed by the acoustic impedance of that particular tissue, depends on the phenomena of interaction between the beam and the material of which the fabric is composed and in particular by the inhomogeneity of the tissue. In fact, a tissue is typically composed of different materials, solids and liquids, with different physical characteristics and therefore different acoustic impedance. At the site where different components of a tissue come in contact, abrupt variations of the acoustic impedance are generated, that is, from the point of view of the propagation of ultrasound, "interfaces" are created (Fig. 2.1). At the level of the interfaces, phenomena of interaction between the ultrasound beam and matter take place, which give reason of the attenuation of the beam.

These phenomena are the following:

- Reflection: that is, the reversal of the direction of propagation so that the ultrasound beam is propagated toward the source of emission. This signal, which is defined echo (return) is called "specular" when the angle of reflection is equal to the incident one and "diffuse" when this angle is different.
- Refraction: at interface, the beam propagates in the same direction but with a different angle from the incident one.
- Transmission: when the acoustic impedance is zero or negligible and the beam conserves both direction and energy.
- Absorption: when the energy of the ultrasound beam is of the order of magnitude of the acoustic impedance and the whole beam fades out, transformed into heat energy [4, 5].

As previously seen, attenuation therefore depends either on the characteristics of the

Fig. 2.1 The surface between two tissues with different acoustic impedance is called interface: when the ultrasound beam crosses an interface, it can be partially or completely reflected, generating an echo

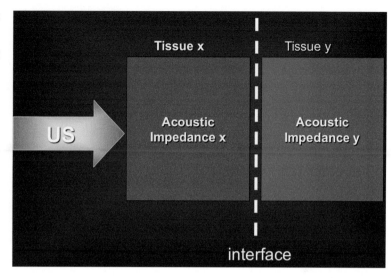

ultrasound beam and on the frequency or the impedance of the acoustic propagation medium. Furthermore, only the reflected component of the ultrasound beam, the returning echo, contributes to the construction of the image; in particular, specular echoes generate the "diagnostic" image and diffuse echoes generate noise (type of artifact) in the image. The amplitude of the returning echo, and therefore its strength, is proportional to the difference in acoustic impedance between adjacent structures, namely, at their interface [6].

Air is characterized by a low propagation velocity (330 m/s) and a very low acoustic impedance (0.0004×10⁶ Rayls, Kg/m²/s). Biological tissues, made largely of water, have similar propagation velocity and acoustic impedance, speed ranging from 1450 m/s for fat to 1580 m/s for the muscle and acoustic impedance from 1.38 to 1.70 10⁶ Rayls (Kg/m²/s) from fat to muscle. Bone tissue is an exception as it has a propagation velocity of 4080 m/s and an acoustic impedance of 7.80 Rayls/kg/m²/s. Therefore in biological tissues, the ultrasound beam may experience both phenomena of refraction and reflection and transmission, and, given the variety of interfaces being penetrated, multiple specular echoes will be produced, at different distances from the emission source. For a given ultrasonic beam at a given frequency and amplitude, the intensity of the produced echoes will depend on the difference in acoustic impedance at the interface and on the distance from the emission source. At the inter-

face with structures characterized by very low (e.g., air in the viscera or lungs) or very high (e.g., bone) acoustic impedance, the sound will be totally reflected, thus generating an intense specular echo. Sound cannot propagate beyond these interfaces, and therefore, an "acoustic vacuum" or posterior shadow cone will be created.

2.5   Ultrasound Generation

In clinical ultrasound, the ultrasonic beam, of which we have described the main features, is generated by the so-called transducers or probes [7].

The ultrasound probes work both as generators of the beam and as receivers of the returning echo and are essentially constituted by an electrical interface and by a set of quartz crystals or of synthetic ceramics capable of generating a "piezoelectric effect." The piezoelectric effect consists in the ability of these crystals to deform when subjected to an appropriate electrical current and to return to their original molecular configuration at the cessation of the electrical impulse (Fig. 2.2). The sudden return to the original configuration causes a resonance phenomenon consisting in a mechanical vibration with the physical characteristics of ultrasound. The beam thus generated can be transmitted only if the probe is acoustically coupled with the tissue to be examined by means of water or of suitable gel, allowing a complete

Fig. 2.2 Ultrasound transducers generate and receive impulses through the piezoelectric properties of crystals: when excited by an electric impulse, they produce an ultrasonic impulse, and vice versa when hit by a returning echo, they generate an electric impulse, which is then converted into a digital image

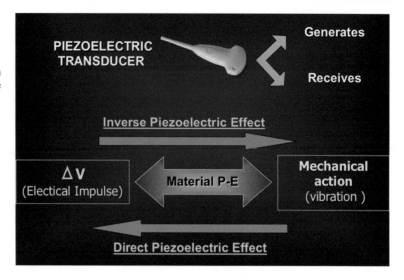

transmission of the beam. This phenomenon is bivalent: in fact, when the crystal is struck by the returning echo, they have the capability to deform and produce an electrical pulse which is proportional to the intensity of the echo. The characteristics of size, physical constitution, and shape of the crystals and the intensity, frequency, and shape of the electrical impulse determine the frequency of functioning of the probe and the characteristics of the ultrasound beam. The probes can be constituted by a single oscillating crystal, therefore capable of producing a conical beam of ultrasound, or by hundreds of crystals arranged next to one another to form different beam shapes. In particular, the most frequently used geometries are linear (crystals arranged on a line, emitting surface flat) and convex (crystals arranged in a semicircle, emitting surface crescent-shaped). A particular configuration of the probe is the sector, having a flat contact surface which is small in size but which is capable of producing a triangular ultrasound beam. The ultrasound beam tends to spread in all directions, so that in order to obtain a preferential direction (along the opening of the probe), it is necessary to use an "acoustic lens" capable to focus the beam in the two dimensions of the space covered by the base of the probe. Actually, the coherence of the beam is maintained up to a distance that depends on the diameter of the crystal (Fresnel zone); deeply in this plane (Fraunhofer zone), the beam tends to diverge. The point of transition between the two areas is the so-called area of focusing of the probe. In modern probes, the use of complex acoustic lenses allows to obtain multiple points of focus. The process of emission of the beam uses the crystal for only 0.1 % of the total time of functioning; the emission phase has a duration in the order of microseconds. For the remaining 99.9 % of the time, the crystal is in the process of reception, or listening, of the returning echoes.

2.6 Signal Reception and Image Formation

The crystals of the probe are capable to transform the returning echoes into electrical impulses [8, 9]. The pulse width is proportional to the amplitude of the returning echoes, and the time elapsed between the emission of the pulse and the returning echo is a measure of the depth at which the interface which produced the echo is positioned. In clinical ultrasound, this estimation is performed by fixing the value of the speed of propagation of ultrasound at 1540 m/s. There are different ways of representing the returning echoes. Historically, the first mode used was the A-mode (amplitude mode) in which the returning echoes were represented as peaks on a line. This mode is monodimensional and does not allow to obtain an image. The B-mode (brightness mode) represents the returning echo as bright spots on a line. The brightness of the point is proportional to the amplitude of the returning echo. This mode is monodimensional, but by obtaining multiple adjacent lines, it is possible to manually build an image. Also if the image thus obtained is processed in a shade of gray proportional to the amplitude of the echo (gray scale), it is possible to enrich the image detail. In the case of the real-time B-mode, the subsequent acquisitions of adjacent scan lines are not performed manually but by means of complex systems of correlation (serial, asynchronous, parallel) of the different groups of crystals that form the probe. In this way, it is possible to obtain two-dimensional images with a temporal frequency (more than 15 images per second) such as to produce a kind of movie with acquisition modalities similar to those of a movie camera. Modern equipment can transform the obtained images in digital images that are generally represented in 256 levels of gray (8-bit depth) and in a 256×356-pixel matrix.

2.7   Characteristics of the Image

The image obtained by ultrasound is an image of reflection, and as such, it is naturally inhomogeneous since deep echoes, coming from the anatomical parts more distant from the probe, are obviously more attenuated. In order to overcome this limitation, devices have systems for selective enhancement of the received signals to compensate for this asymmetrical attenuation. The TGC (time gain compensation) allows precisely to selectively amplify the late (and therefore more attenuated) echoes [10]. In general, the signal of the hepatic and splenic parenchyma serves as reference parameter. We will refer to the word isoechoic for echoes of intensity comparable to that of these reference parenchyma and hyper-

echoic or hypoechoic for those of higher or lower intensity (Fig. 2.3). It is understandable that this classification, albeit universal, is highly operator dependent. Considered anechoic is everything that does not produce a returning echo as, for example, the fluid contained in a simple cyst (Fig. 2.4). A key feature of the image is spatial resolution. It can be distinguished in axial resolution (Fig. 2.5), along the axis of propagation of ultrasound and lateral resolution (Fig. 2.6), perpendicular to it. The axial resolution depends on the frequency in a direct relation, and its theoretical maximum value cannot be greater than half the wavelength of the beam. Therefore, probes with greater frequency allow to obtain higher resolutions although they are limited by the fact that their penetration capacity is proportionately lower. Lateral resolution depends on the size of the crystals. Even in this case, smaller crystals provide greater resolution at the expense of the capacity of penetration.

2.8   Artifacts in Ultrasound Imaging

Ultrasounds present some typical artifacts that can generate false information but sometimes are useful to the correct interpretation of the image [11, 12]. Therefore, they will be divided into useful and harmful.

Useful artifacts are the following:

• Posterior wall enhancement (Fig. 2.7): it takes place rearward formations of fluid such as cysts and derives from the fact that the ultrasound beam through the cyst is not attenuated contrary to what happens to the contiguous beams. Therefore at a level deeper than the cyst, it generates echoes with a greater amplitude than the adjacent beams, especially at the hard interface between fluid and solid. It may be useful to differentiate a liquid structure from a highly hypoechoic but solid one.
• Shadow cone (Fig. 2.8): it is generated at the interface between structures with marked difference of acoustic impedance, generally between

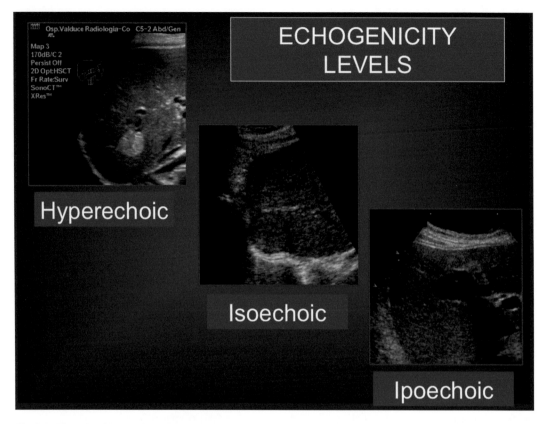

Fig. 2.3 Three focal hepatic lesions are reported, with different echogenicity compared to normal hepatic parenchyma: hyperechoic, isoechoic, and hypoechoic

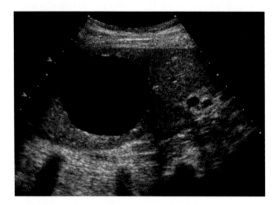

Fig. 2.4 Fluid collections are completely anechoic, not having interfaces nor texture

tissues and bone or calcified structures (such as kidney stones). It may be useful to identify a kidney or choledocic stone or parenchymal calcification. In the case of air, the shadow cone is not absolute because phenomena of reverber-

ation are generally present as well. In this case, the reflection is so radical as to produce a reflected secondary beam which is then reflected secondarily from the surface of the transducer and is represented (since it is late) as a linear echo below the shadow cone.

- Edge shadowing: it appears as a thin hypoechoic line that extends from the side wall of an anechoic yet provided with wall, for clarity structure (such as the aorta) when this is insonated transversely. It is useful, in the case of the aorta, to improve the accuracy of measurement (being a very obvious echo).
- Comet-tail artifact (Fig. 2.9): it is a particular reverberation artifact which is generated by multiple reflections between the front and rear wall of small calcifications. It depends on the size, shape, and composition of microcalcifications. It can be useful in recognizing them.

Fig. 2.5 Axial resolution: the ability of the system to differentiate between two structures that lie at different depths along the axis of the ultrasound beam and depends upon pulse length.
L refers to the pulse lenght, *A* and *B* represent 2 echo generating structures, *d1* is the distance between these 2 structures. If d is >1/2 wavelength, the 2 structures will be identified as 2 distinct structures; if d is <1/2 wavelength, the 2 structures will be identified as one

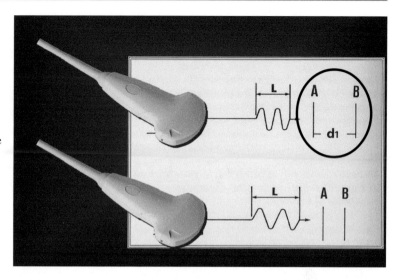

Fig. 2.6 Lateral resolution: the ability of the system to differentiate between two structures that lie at the same depth perpendicular to the axis of the ultrasound beam and depends upon pulse width

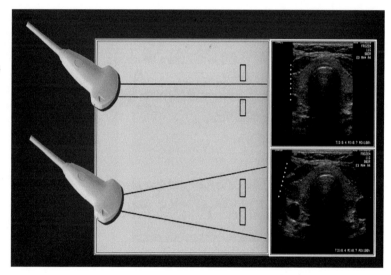

Harmful artifacts are essentially reverberation artifacts that are created at the interface of structures with large difference in acoustic impedance, generally structures containing air. As already explained in these cases, secondary reflected beams can be generated and interpreted as real, and this can determine erroneous topographic interpretations (diaphragm position, reflection of hyperechoic lesions of the liver above the diaphragm) or even create nonexisting lesions (Fig. 2.10). They are usually found beneath the diaphragm domes.

2.9   The Biological Effects of Ultrasound

In principle, both very high and very low sound frequencies can cause damage. We have seen that the mechanical energy transmitted via ultrasound can be absorbed in the form of heat. In addition, mechanical vibration can cause rupture of ties or cavitation (i.e., the formation of vacuoles) in intracellular compartment. These phenomena, however, are strongly dependent on the energy of the beam and on the

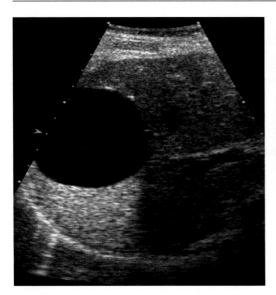

Fig. 2.7 Going through a fluid collection (completely anechoic), the attenuation phenomena is reduced; therefore, the tissues posterior to an anechoic structure will have an augmented echogenicity

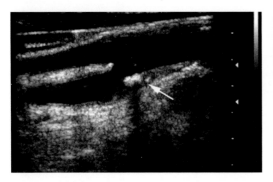

Fig. 2.8 Posterior shadows are generated by anatomical structures with elevated acoustic impedance that determines a complete reflection of the ultrasound beam. The image shows an ultrasound view of the carotid bifurcation; the hyperechoic structure indicated by the *arrow* is a fibrous plaque, generating a posterior shadow

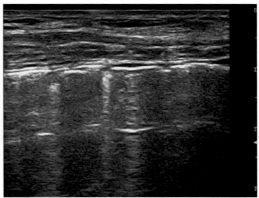

Fig. 2.9 Pulmonary comet tail: thin hyperechoic vertical lines that go deep in the lung parenchyma from the lung/pleural interface. They correspond to the high acoustic impedance between thickened interlobular fibrous tissues in pulmonary fibrosis

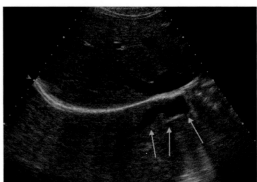

Fig. 2.10 When a structure is in close proximity to a curved interface with high reflection (diaphragm, bladder), it can be visualized in its real position and on the opposite side of the interface: these are multiple reflections between the surface and the anatomical structure itself, with a dilation of the time that the echo needs to reach back the ultrasound probe. The picture shows an ultrasound image of the liver, with vascular hypoechoic structures and a hyperechoic structure (diaphragm). The *arrows* point to an artifactual image, which is generated by a mirror-effect between the vascular hepatic structure and the diaphragm

time of application of ultrasound and require, in order to occur, exposures of the order of seconds. We have seen that the emission time of a crystal is of the order of microseconds, and the energies used by the ultrasound in diagnostic medicine are extremely low (no more than 50 mW/cm²). The biological hazards in the diagnostic field are therefore null [13].

References

1. Edmonds PD (1981) Methods of experimental physics, vol 19, Ultrasonic. Academic Press, 111 Fifth Avenue, New York, New York, 10003
2. Richardson EG (1952) Ultrasonic physics. Elsevier Publishing Company, 52 Vanderbilt Avenue, New York 17, N.Y.

3. Crawford AE (1955) Ultrasonic engineering. Butterworths Scientific Publications, London
4. Pisani R, Liboni W (1999) Principi fisici degli ultrasuoni. In: Rabbia C, De Lucchi R, Cirillo R (eds) Ecodoppler vascolare. Edizioni Minerva Medica, Torino
5. Dickinson RJ (1986) Refl ection and scattering. In: Hill CR (ed) Physical principles of medical ultrasonics. Ellis Horwood, Chichester
6. Duck FA (1990) Physical properties of tissue – a comprehensive reference book. Academic, London
7. Carpenter DA (1980) Ultrasonic trasducer. Clin Diagn Ultrasound 5:31/39
8. Whittingham TA (1999) An overview of digital technology in ultrasonic imaging. Technology section 2: digital technology. Eur Radiol 9:S307–S311
9. Whittingham TA (1999) Broadband transducers. Technology section 1: new transducers. Eur Radiol 9:S298–S303
10. Taylor KJW, Mc Cready VR (1976) A clinical evaluation of gray scale ultrasonography. Br J Radiol 49:244/252
11. Laing FC (1983) Commonly encountered artifacts in clinical ultrasound. Semin Ultrasound 4:27–43
12. Sommer FG, Filly RA, Minton MJ (1979) Acoustic shadowing due to refractive and reflective effects. Am J Roentgenol 132:973–977
13. Baker ML, Dalrymple GV (1978) Biological effects of diagnostic ultrasound: a review. Radiology 126: 479–483

Part II

B-Mode Ultrasound

Ultrasound System Setup and General Semeiology

3

Luca Maria Sconfienza, Giovanni Mauri, and Francesco Secchi

3.1 Introduction

As reported in the previous chapters, ultrasound imaging is based on a relatively simple principle, i.e., the reflection of ultrasound waves by the biologic tissues. On the other hand, late-end ultrasound systems are very sophisticated machines that need to be set up carefully to achieve good diagnostic performances. The setup process is usually performed by the vendor once the system is installed, according to the needed clinical applications. In daily practice, however, there is a number of different parameters that can be adjusted to optimize the ultrasound image.

L.M. Sconfienza, MD, PhD (✉)
Institute of Radiology, Università degli Studi di Milano, San Donato Milanese, Italy

Radiology Unit, IRCCS Policlinico San Donato, San Donato Milanese, Italy
e-mail: io@lucasconfienza.it

G. Mauri, MD
Department of Radiology, Policlinico San Donato, San Donato Milanese (Milano), Italy

Department of Interventional Radiology, European Institute of Oncology, Milano, Italy

F. Secchi, MD
Department of Biomedical Sciences for Health, Università degli Studi di Milano, Milan, Italy

3.2 The Console of the Ultrasound System

As obvious, each vendor produces ultrasound systems that differ in terms of many features, including the external design and, occasionally, the names given to the various commands and tools. However, the main commands are generally easily and directly accessible from the console (Fig. 3.1). Also, note that many recent ultrasound systems are provided with touch screen displays where the advanced tools pertinent to the ongoing examinations are summarized.

3.2.1 Trackball

It is a sort of a "reverse" edition of a mouse that is normally used on personal computers. Rotating the ball makes the pointer moving on the monitor to perform different operations: indicating, measuring a lesion, set markers, and so on. In some systems, it is also used to set the correct depth of the beam focus. The trackball is usually surrounded by a number of buttons (in the system displayed in Fig. 3.1, there are four buttons surrounding the trackball) that can be used to select functions, similar to what happens for conventional mouses. While buttons on mouses usually have fixed functions (i.e., left button, select; right button, context menu), these buttons

F. Prada et al. (eds.), *Intraoperative Ultrasound (IOUS) in Neurosurgery: From Standard B-mode to Elastosonography*, DOI 10.1007/978-3-319-25268-1_3

are totally programmable and can be used for different actions. Trackball is indicated as #1 on Fig. 3.1.

3.2.2 Depth

This command is used to set the optimal image depth. All probes are set to a specific standard image depth. According to the depth of the lesion/organ to assess, the image can be made deeper or more superficial to achieve optimal visualization of the whole target. Increasing the depth, the ultrasound image will penetrate more in the tissues and the image will result smaller. Reducing the depth, the ultrasound image will be reduced to the most superficial tissues and will result bigger; however, spatial resolution is also reduced and the image may be unsatisfactory. This command should not be confused with the zoom tool, which is used to magnify a specific area of interest, regardless of the depth. Figure 3.2 shows the same structure with two different depth settings.

3.2.3 Focus

Focus management may be embedded in the trackball (see above) or done with a separate command. Focus should be carefully placed in the center of the imaged area to achieve optimal visibility. Note that the number of focal point can be varied (usually up to four), using a different command. Examples of correct and incorrect focus positioning are shown in Fig. 3.3.

3.2.4 Gain

This tool is very similar to a control for image brightness. Essentially, it controls the amplifica-

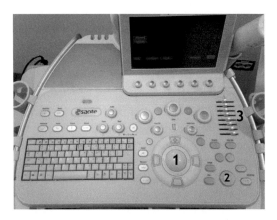

Fig. 3.1 Console of a commercial ultrasound system. A large number of commands can be seen, which are usually arranged differently among various vendors. However, three main commands are usually very similar regardless the brand. *1* trackball surrounded by four buttons, *2* freeze button, *3* time gain control setting

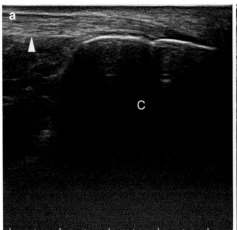
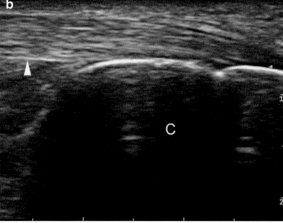

Fig. 3.2 Two different depth setting. (**a**) The image is set very deep. The Achilles tendon (*arrowheads*) is seen relatively small but spatial definition is good. *C* calcaneus. (**b**) The image is set very superficial. The Achilles tendon is magnified but spatial definition is relatively poor

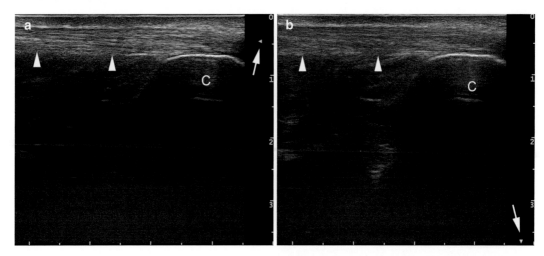

Fig. 3.3 (**a**) Correct and (**b**) incorrect focus positioning in a longitudinal scan of the Achilles tendon. (**a**) The tendon (*arrowheads*) has well defined margins, particularly the deeper, and nicely seen fibrillar echotexture. The focus is indicated by a small side triangle (*arrow*) and is correctly positioned at the level of the tendon. *C* calcaneus. (**b**) The focus is positioned very deep (*arrow*) and the tendon is poorly seen. Note the ill-definition of the deep margin and of the fibrillar echotexture

tion of electronic signal produced by ultrasound waves. It controls the strength of the echoes that are received from the probe. From a practical point of view, gain increase will result in a brighter image. Different gain settings are shown in Fig. 3.4.

3.2.5   Time Gain Control (TGC)

In the previous chapters, it has been reported that ultrasound beam progressively attenuates as it progresses into the body tissues. TGC allows for correcting the sensitivity of the ultrasound system at different depth, thus compensating signal loss in deeper portions of larger organs (e.g., liver, brain, etc.). As can be seen, this command is composed by a series of sliders that can be set independently, thus allowing for optimization of the gain in every single layer. As depth of different layers on ultrasound image depends on the time needed by the ultrasound beam to go forth and back, this tool is named *time gain control*. TGC command is indicated as #3 on Fig. 3.1.

3.2.6   Frequency

In the previous chapters, it has been reported that the higher the frequency, the higher the spatial resolution and the lower the penetration of the ultrasound beam. Conversely, the lower the frequency, the lower the spatial resolution and the higher the penetration of beam. The frequency is an intrinsic property of each probe and cannot be changed. However, modern probes are called multifrequency, which means they have a spectrum of frequencies that can be used for imaging. This tool allows for adjusting the frequency of the probe within a specific range, thus resulting in more detailed or more penetrating images. Different frequency settings are shown in Fig. 3.5.

3.2.7   Freeze

This is probably the most frequently used command and usually has the biggest button on the console. Being ultrasonography a real-time imaging modality, it shows images in motion. This command is used to fix a single frame on the

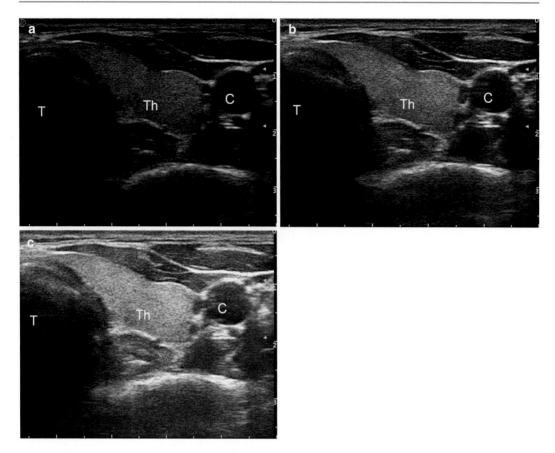

Fig. 3.4 Different gain settings. On the same axial scan of the left lobe of the thyroid (*Th*), the gain is set at (**a**) low, (**b**) intermediate, and (**c**) high level. In (**a**), gain is too low, as contrast between the thyroid and the surrounding muscles is poor. In (**c**), gain is too high, as the carotid artery (*C*) seems to contain some hyperechoic material. In (**b**), gain is set at an intermediate, correct level. *T* trachea

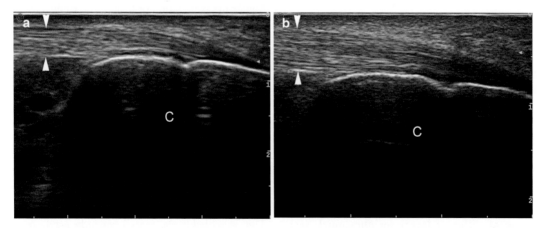

Fig. 3.5 Effect of frequency variation using two different high-resolution broadband linear array probes. In (**a**), the Achilles tendon (*arrowheads*) is imaged using a 6–13 MHz probe. The fibrillar echotexture can be seen and beam penetration is reasonably deep. Here, the image is cut at 3-cm depth. *C* calcaneus. In (**b**), the tendon is imaged using a 6–18 MHz probe. The fibrillar echotexture is seen in higher detail, resembling histological section; however, image depth is as limited as 2 cm from the skin surface

Fig. 3.6 Use of calipers to measure the right thyroid lobe (*Th*). Anterior-posterior diameter is indicated by caliper #1 (*arrows*), while medial-lateral diameter is indicated by caliper #2 (*arrowheads*). Measures are reported on the side of the image (*curved arrow*). *T* trachea, *C* carotid

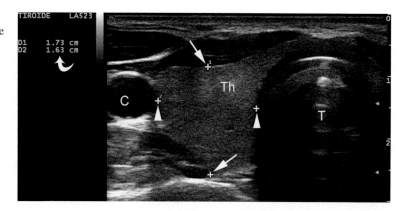

screen. While the image is frozen, the operator can perform a number of actions (e.g., place annotations, measure diameters, store and print, etc.). Freeze command is indicated as #2 on Fig. 3.1.

3.2.8   Caliper

This tool is used to measure a distance (e.g., the diameter of a lesion, the length of an organ, etc.). When this tool is selected, the pointer usually becomes a small cross. The cross is placed on one side of the lesion and one of the buttons of the trackball is pressed. Then, using the trackball, the cross is moved on the other side of the lesion and the button is clicked again. The system usually traces a line between the two marks and the measure is displayed over/aside the image. Note that, in most system, when the caliper button is pressed, a number of different measurement options can be selected (e.g., area, angle, etc.), usually from a side menu. Use of calipers is shown in Fig. 3.6.

3.3   General Semeiology

Being ultrasound an imaging modality mainly based on gray-scale images, a tissue or an organ can be brighter or darker of another. The intrinsic brightness of a tissue or organ is generally known as *echogenicity*. In conventional ultrasound terminology, the echogenicity of a tissue should be compared to that of a different surrounding structure (e.g., a muscle when dealing with the thy-

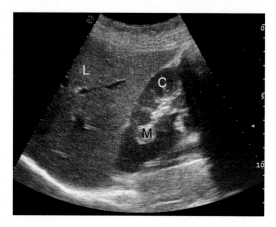

Fig. 3.7 Different echogenicities of solid organs in the abdomen. The renal medulla (*M*) is very bright, the liver (*L*) has intermediate brightness, and the renal cortex (*C*) is dark. It can also be said that the liver parenchyma is hyperechoic compared to the renal cortex (this is a cases of mild hepatic steatosis). Also, the renal medulla is more hyperechoic than the liver

roid, the right kidney when dealing with the liver, etc), stating that "it is brighter than…" or "it is darker than…" (Fig. 3.7). However, in current clinical practice, the terms that are reported below are generally used as synonyms of bright and dark.

3.3.1   Hyperechoic

A tissue that is brighter than another (e.g., the subcutaneous fat is hyperechoic compared to the underlying muscles). In general, it is used as a synonym of bright.

3.3.2 Isoechoic

A tissue that is as bright as another (e.g., the kidney cortex isoechoic to the normal liver parenchyma). In general, it is used to report the appearance of a lesion (e.g., a liver nodule that is isoechoic to the surrounding parenchyma).

3.3.3 Hypoechoic

A tissue that is darker than another (e.g., the muscles are hypoechoic compared to the overlying subcutaneous fat). In general, it is used as a synonym of dark.

3.3.4 Anechoic

As ultrasound images are the graphical representation of ultrasound waves reflecting on tissue interfaces, purely fluid structures or collections have no signal at all (i.e., are totally anechoic), as the beam has no interfaces to reflect on. For this reason, areas in which the ultrasound beam is not reflected are called anechoic (without echoes). Absence of echoes is shown in Fig. 3.8.

As reported in the previous chapters, the ultrasound image is strictly related to the ratio between beam that crosses interfaces between the different layers of biologic tissues and beam that is reflected. Also, within the single layer of tissue, there are interfaces that further contribute to determine the intrinsic appearance of an organ, generally known as *echotexture*. The echotexture

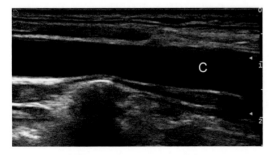

Fig. 3.8 Ultrasound scan of the common carotid artery (*C*). No interfaces are present within the vessel, as it contains fluid. Thus, the artery appears totally dark

of a biologic tissue strongly reflects the histological arrangement of the tissue itself. Different types of echotextures are:

3.3.5 Solid

This echotexture is generally typical of parenchymal organs, such as the liver, the thyroid, the spleen, and also the brain. The ultrasound image has the typical appearance of a homogeneous, finely granular tissue. Examples of solid echotexture are shown in Fig. 3.7.

3.3.6 Liquid

It is basically a synonym of anechoic. Examples of purely fluid areas are the bladder, the arteries and the veins, and also the brain ventricles. When fluid in a collection is not purely anechoic, the composition may be different from normal hyaline fluids (e.g., pus collection). An example of fluid collection is shown in Fig. 3.8.

3.3.7 Mixed

When areas of hyperechoic and hypoechoic tissue, or fluid and solid tissues, coexist in the same tissue, organ, or lesion, the echotexture is defined as mixed (e.g., a mixed nodule of the thyroid, in which solid tissue and cystic areas coexist in the same lesion). This type of echotexture is not generally typical of normal organs. A mixed thyroid nodule is shown in Fig. 3.9.

3.3.8 Multilayered

Muscle bellies are made by muscular fascicles interspersed with perimysial septa. This arrangement is seen on ultrasound as a typical hypo-hyperechoic multilayered texture on a long-axis scan. On a short axis, a kind of geometrical appearance can be appreciated. Multilayered echotexture is shown in Fig. 3.10.

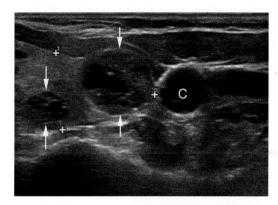

Fig. 3.9 Mixed thyroid nodules (*arrows*). Note the coexistence of solid and liquid areas in the same nodule. *C* carotid artery

3.3.9 Fascicular

Peripheral nerves are made by nerve fascicle interspersed with fat. On a long-axis scan, they appear like hypo-hyperechoic striated bands running between muscles and under the retinacula. On a short-axis scan, they have a typical honeycomb appearance. Example of fascicular echotexture is shown in Fig. 3.11.

3.3.10 Fibrillar

Tendons are made of highly reflective collagen fibers packed together. Thus, they appear as

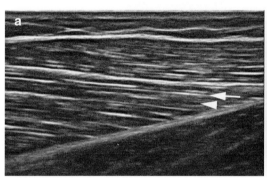
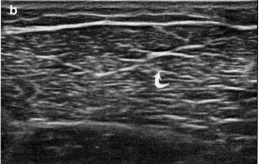

Fig. 3.10 Multilayered appearance of muscle tissue on (**a**) long- and (**b**) short-axis scan. (**a**) On a long-axis scan, the regular pattern of hyperechoic perimysial septa (*arrow*) and hypoechoic muscle fascicles (*arrowhead*) can be seen. (**b**) On a short-axis scan, the typical mosaic appearance can be seen (*curved arrow*)

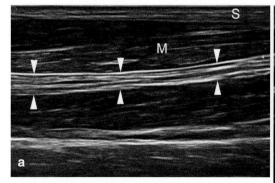
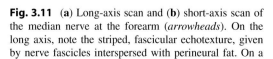
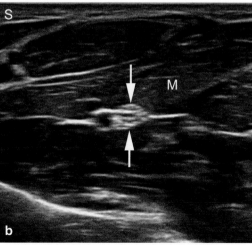

Fig. 3.11 (**a**) Long-axis scan and (**b**) short-axis scan of the median nerve at the forearm (*arrowheads*). On the long axis, note the striped, fascicular echotexture, given by nerve fascicles interspersed with perineural fat. On a short axis, the typical honeycomb appearance can be clearly seen (*arrows*). The surrounding muscles (*M*) are hypoechoic compared to the nerve. The subcutaneous tissue (*S*) is hyperechoic compared to muscles

Fig. 3.12 (**a**) Long- and (**b**) short-axis scan of the Achilles tendon (*arrowheads*). On the long axis, note the typical hyperechoic fibrillar echotexture that differentiates this structure from nerves (see Fig. 3.11). On the short axis, the tendon has a fine salt-and-pepper echotexture

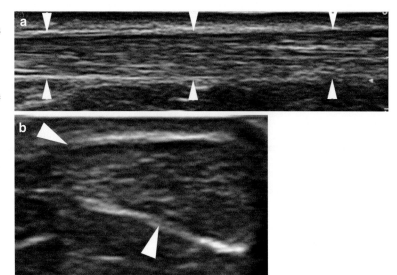

Fig. 3.13 Hyper-reflective surface of the radius (*arrowheads*). The ultrasound beam is almost completely reflected by the bone cortex. The signal seen below the cortex (*asterisks*) is an artifact

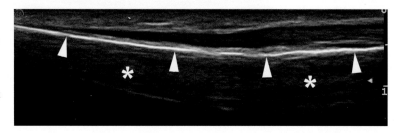

strongly hyperechoic fibrillar bands between muscles. Example of fibrillar echotexture is shown in Fig. 3.12.

3.3.11 Highly Reflective

Ultrasound has two bitter enemies: the bone and air. Both reflect a high amount of the incident ultrasound beam (i.e., the bone reflects about 45 % and air reflects about 99.95 % of the incident ultrasound beam). This explains why coupling gel is needed to fill the air gap between the probe and the surface of the organs, image of gas-containing structures is largely unfeasible (e.g., lung, bowel, etc.), or scanning the brain without opening the skull is not possible. Highly reflective appearance of the bone cortex is shown in Fig. 3.13.

Further readings

Støylen A. Basic ultrasound, echocardiography and Doppler for clinicians. http://folk.ntnu.no/stoylen/strainrate/Ultrasound/. Accessed 30 June 2015

Wikiradiography. http://www.wikiradiography.net/page/Ultrasound+Physics. Accessed 30 June 2015

Xu D. Optimizing an ultrasound image. http://www.nysora.com/mobile/regional-anesthesia/foundations-of-us-guided-nerve-blocks-techniques/3085-optimizing-an-ultrasound-image.html. Accessed 30 June 2015

UCLA team. Regional anesthesia, basic principles. http://www.usra.ca/tissueecho.php. Accessed 30 June 2015

Echographic Brain Semeiology and Topographic Anatomy According to Surgical Approaches

4

Francesco Prada, Massimiliano Del Bene,
Alessandro Moiraghi, and Francesco DiMeco

4.1   Introduction

Intraoperative imaging is nowadays of routine use in almost every neurosurgical procedure. The main tools are represented by neuro-navigation systems (NN), which are based on preoperative imaging; consequently they cannot describe the changes that occur during surgery [1–4]. The necessity to not rely only on preoperative imaging leaded to introduce intraoperative imaging such as magnetic resonance imaging (MRI), computed tomography (CT), and fluorescence imaging. Each of these techniques suffers from major limitation: MRI and CT are not real time, representing only the situation at the time of image acquisition, while fluorescence is not an anatomical imaging modality because it can be observed only on the surface of the surgical bed [5–7].

Intraoperative ultrasound (IOUS) provides real-time direct visualization of the explored area. Its use in neurosurgery has been first described in 1978 by Reid [8]. Over the years a lot of neurosurgical procedures were reported to be guided by IOUS: lesion localization in the brain and spine, guidance of surgical resection, catheter placement, aspiration of abscess, decompression control in Chiari I malformation, and others [9–15]. Theoretically IOUS is particularly indicated in neurosurgery. Brain parenchyma has specific viscoelastic features that permit exceptional US propagation also because US beam is not attenuated by interposed skin and subcutaneous connective tissues [16]. Moreover IOUS is truly real time and characterized by a superb temporal and spatial resolution [17]. These aspects permit to visualize the real surgical-anatomical scenario during the entire surgical procedure and, in particular condition, to operate under direct IOUS control.

Notwithstanding that, currently, IOUS is not widespread in neurosurgery. This is mainly due to the fact that IOUS is not a routinely diagnostic tool and there is a lack in the brain and spinal US semeiotics and topographic anatomy: consequently most of neurosurgons are not familiar whit US. In particular, brain and spine imaging is traditionally performed following the three panoramic orthogonal planes of MRI and CT (coronal, sagittal, and axial). On the

F. Prada, MD (✉) • M. Del Bene • A. Moiraghi
Department of Neurosurgery, Fondazione IRCCS
Istituto Neurologico C. Besta,
via Celoria 11, Milan 20133, Italy
e-mail: francesco.prada@istituto-besta.it

F. DiMeco
Department of Neurosurgery, Fondazione IRCCS
Istituto Neurologico C. Besta,
via Celoria 11, Milan 20133, Italy

Department of Neurological Surgery, Johns Hopkins
Medical School, Baltimore, MD, USA

© Springer International Publishing Switzerland 2016
F. Prada et al. (eds.), *Intraoperative Ultrasound (IOUS) in Neurosurgery:
From Standard B-mode to Elastosonography*, DOI 10.1007/978-3-319-25268-1_4

other hand, IOUS generates an unusual tomographic representation of what is visible in the insonation plan, that is, consequence of probe positioning and surgical approaches: the orientation is usually rotated and it is sectorial and generally in an unusual plan. Additionally, IOUS is extremely demanding because of the number of parameters and settings of a US device and the various phenomena that take place during surgery and change the US semeiotics. IOUS is therefore considered an operator-dependant technique with a steep learning curve [13, 15, 18, 19]. Therefore in the past, also given the low spatial resolution, other intraoperative imaging techniques have been preferred to IOUS, which remained far from being a standard tool. With the recent advancement in spatial and temporal resolution, along with additional aid in imaging interpretation such as fusion imaging and CEUS, IOUS is becoming more exploited. However, general rules have to be applied, in order to properly perform an IOUS evaluation and obtain reproducible information. In this chapter we will try to standardize the intraoperative settings for IOUS application in neurosurgery, together with main semiotics findings.

4.2   IOUS Equipment, Operative Setting

4.2.1   IOUS Equipment

In our institution we use a last generation US device (MyLab, Esaote, Italy) predisposed for contrast-enhanced ultrasound, elastosonography, and fusion imaging between preoperative imaging and IOUS for virtual navigation, using a dedicated virtual navigation software (MedCom GmbH, Germany). Anyhow, in general a last generation portable US device could be sufficient. We generally employ a linear array multi-frequency (3–11 MHz) probe with trapezoidal view for both superficial and deep-seated lesions and also for Doppler execution (Fig. 4.1). For

superficial lesions, a linear array high-frequency probe (10–22 MHz) might be used (Fig. 4.1) [19]. A small micro-convex multi-frequency probe can be used for small craniotomies or to explore surgical cavities.

The physics of echo generation from US explains that the higher the US frequency, the higher the spatial resolution, but lower is the penetration, and vice versa. For this aspect, it is really practical to have multi-frequency probes that can cover the most used frequency both for depth and superficial lesions.

4.2.2   Operative Setting

The operating room must be large enough to permit the US device to be located on the left of the first surgeon. The US device must be prepared to be used by the operator during the surgery, and the user interface (touch screen monitor and keyboard) must be accessible to the operator (e.g., covered by sterile transparent drape) (Fig. 4.2). The probe is wrapped in plastic sterile sheet together with sterile US-compatible gel. It is mandatory that the surgeon can easily set the US device during all the surgery (Fig. 4.2).

The patient must be positioned, when possible, to allow the surgical field to be horizontal in order to be filled by saline solution for best US coupling. The craniotomy must be large enough to house the probe (maximum diameter: 3.5 cm) and permitting its free tilting and orientation (Figs. 4.2, 4.3, 4.4).

4.3   IOUS Exam

Main aim of intraoperative B-mode study is to visualize the entire lesion and its relationships with the healthy neurovascular structures/brain parenchyma. In order to do this, it is essential to use the correct magnification power, and in some cases, a gel-pad spacer can be useful. It is of help to perform the first scan with a wide field of view,

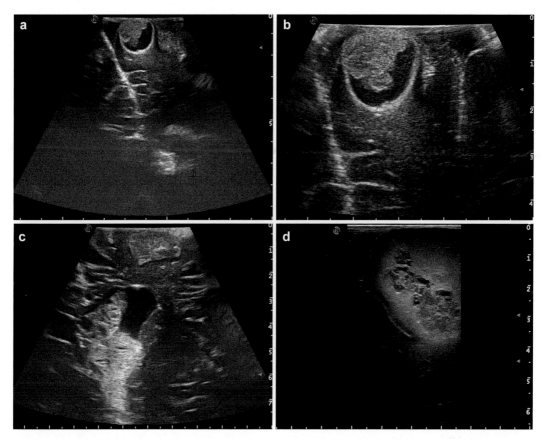

Fig. 4.1 Magnification power and probe frequency. First scan must be performed with a wide field of view to visualize the main target along with its surrounding structures (**a**). Then the magnification power must be increased to better understand lesion morphology and surrounding tissue (**b**). The higher the US frequency, the higher the spatial resolution, but the lower is the penetration (**d**), and vice versa (**c**). A multifrequency probe can cover the most used frequency both for deep and superficial lesions

adjusting depth and angle of insonation, in order to visualize the main target along with its surrounding structures. Then the lesion should be examined with greater detail, reducing the depth, to better analyze its structures and surrounding tissues (Fig. 4.1).

The main parameters that have to be adjusted and allow to correctly visualize the target according to changing in depth and width of field are frequency, power, and focus. It is also of great help to prepare different presets for different lesions.

The first B-mode scan must be executed before opening the dura mater and later on, during surgery, every time it is needed, and at the end of tumor resection to check for potential residual mass (Fig. 4.2).

We believe that the methodology of the exam should be standardized as much as possible, especially for those users not accustomed to echo-tomographic images.

The two-dimensional basal scan comprises two types of acquisition:

- Orthogonal scan: the probe is positioned in the center of the craniotomy. The lesion has to be visualized on two orthogonal planes to obtain

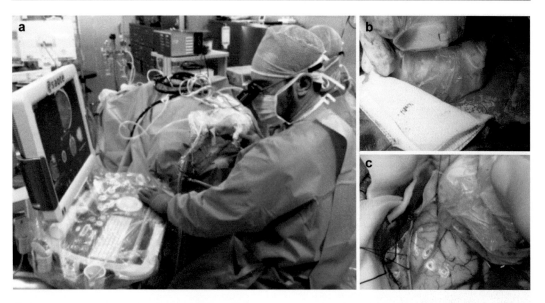

Fig. 4.2 Intraoperative setting. (**a**) The US machine is placed on the left hand side of the patient and the keyboard is wrapped in a plastic sterile cover to allow the surgeon direct access to all commands throughout the procedure. Main parameters to be changed are frequency, depth, and gain. Other tools are Doppler, contrast, and elastography. Through direct control of the machine, it is also possible to review the acquired images and further define the surgical strategy. The probe is wrapped in plastic sterile sheath together with sterile US gel and it is used to perform a first scan on intact dura mater (**b**) and multiple scans during surgery (**c**)

a complete overview and its major relationships (Fig. 4.3).
- Probe tilting and shifting to perform a detailed study of the region of interest and to create a three-dimensional visualization of the lesion (Fig. 4.4).

4.3.1 Orthogonal Scan

- Place the probe in the center of the craniotomy with the probe indicator oriented upward, toward patient's front, or toward patient's left side (depending on approach, craniotomy site and patient positioning).
- Depending on the craniotomy site, it will be possible to scan the lesion only on two orthogonal planes (Fig. 4.3):
  - Sagittal–axial (e.g., in case of frontal approach)
  - Sagittal–coronal (e.g., in case of coronal/parietal approach)
  - Coronal–axial (e.g., in case of pterional approach)

- Be sure to identify the lesion, its relationships and other relevant structures/landmarks. The orthogonal scan should first be performed with a large depth (at least 7–8 cm.), surpassing the midline, in order to evaluate the whole of the lesion along with its surrounding anatomical landmarks. Then it is possible to zoom on the lesion to evaluate its borders.

4.3.2 Probe Tilting and Shifting

- Tilting the probe on two orthogonal axes, it is possible to enlarge the field of view also below the craniotomy margins. This feature permits to find a greater number of landmarks and as a consequence to understand insonation plane orientation and US semeiotics. Moreover, in case of large lesions, all the margins became examinable.

If the operculum is large enough, it is possible to shift the probe on two orthogonal axes in order

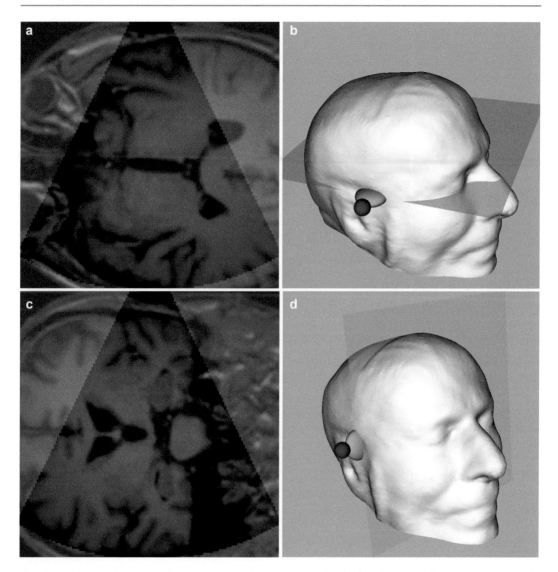

Fig. 4.3 Orthogonal scans. US probe on a three-dimensional model (**b, d**) and corresponding planes of insonation reconstructed from an MRI (**a, c**). As mentioned in the text, with each approach it is possible to perform a scan only on two orthogonal planes and their various declination. However it is not possible to obtain images along the plane that is perpendicular to the plane of the probe or parallel to main axis of the craniotomy (sagittal plane as in this case)

to complete the study, obtaining a mental tridimensional reconstruction of the volume (Fig. 4.4).

The variation of the probe's position should be done with slow movements in a standardized way:

- From left to right for the sagittal plan
- From anterior to posterior for the coronal plan
- From top to bottom for the axial plan

Using the two-dimensional tomographic real-time visual information integrated with those provided by the hand movement and position of the probe in the space, the operator should try to create a three-dimensional mental reconstruction of the region of interest. If available an automatic three-dimensional reconstruction might be used. In some cases (e.g., posterior fossa, spinal surgery, keyhole

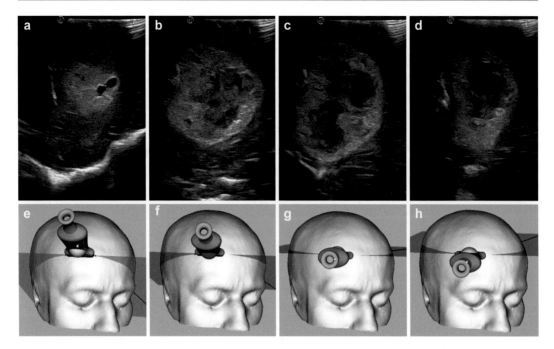

Fig. 4.4 Probe tilting. US images of a right frontal metastasis, obtained tilting the probe (**a**–**d**). In the lower panel a three-dimensional model represent the corresponding probe orientation (**e**–**h**)

approaches, etc.) it is not possible to tilt and shift the probe because of the scarce space in the surgical field.

4.3.2.1 IOUS Cerebral Semeiotics

Normal ultrasound appearance of major structures and practical anatomical landmarks (Fig. 4.5):

- Hyperechoic structures: skull, vessels wall, choroid plexuses, arachnoidal folds, ependyma, dural fold, brain-lesion interface
- Hypoechoic structures: cerebrospinal fluid, ventricles, connective fibers
- Isoechoic structures: brain parenchyma

Normal brain parenchyma is generally homogeneous and iso-hypoechoic. The surfaces of the cortical gyri appear moderately hyperechoic for a depth of a few millimeters, corresponding to the gray matter, while the lobar white matter is more hyperechoic due to presence of vascular channels. Large connective structures such as the cor-

pus callosum are hypoechoic. The basal ganglia appear slightly hyperechoic, probably because of higher vasculature and presence of microcalcifications (Fig. 4.5).

Cerebral ventricles appear hypoechoic and typically surrounded by a thin hyperechoic rim, corresponding to the ependymal wall, which determines a strong interface between the parenchyma and CSF. Choroid plexuses are highly hyperechoic and can be visualized in the ventricles, representing one of the most reliable landmarks together with main dural folds. The falx cerebri and tentorium cerebelli appear as thin, linear, and hyperechoic structures. Vessel walls usually appear hyperechoic surrounding the hypoechoic lumen; this feature gives to main arteries the typical rail aspect (Fig. 4.5).

In most cases, contrast between tumor and healthy structures is sufficient to distinguish tumor-brain interface, also in case of perilesional edema. Acute edema is generally hypoechoic than tumors, whereas chronic edema can be iso- or hyperechoic.

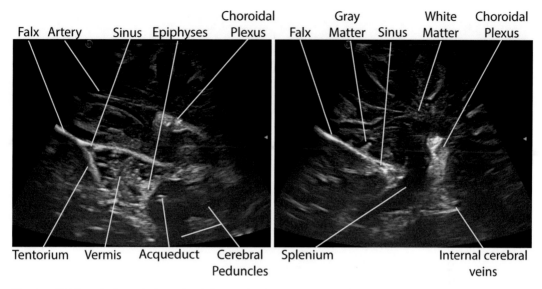

Fig. 4.5 IOUS cerebral semeiotics and main landmarks along the two possible orthogonal planes in a parietal approach

Most primary or metastatic brain tumors are hyperechoic relative to the surrounding normal brain parenchyma and also to edematous tissues (hyperechoic). Some lesion may present extremely echogenic portions, as for calcified nodules in meningioma, whereas cystic and necrotic regions appear as hypoechoic fluid-filled cavities that can show back reinforcement phenomenon. On the other hand, highly infiltrative lesions such as low-grade gliomas have not well-defined margins, in particular in case of surrounding edema [20].

It is mandatory to remember that the IOUS semeiotics is not static but dynamic. Surgical manipulation of tumor and brain leads to a drop in diagnostic accuracy, mainly due to the appearance of artifacts [18, 21]. Blood clots and hemostatic materials within the surgical cavity are hyperechoic and create an acoustic shadow that does not permit study of the cavity wall to find the tumor-brain interface.

Moreover, the surrounding parenchyma tends to become edematous because of the surgical maneuvers; this feature makes the tumor and brain contrast less clear [18].

All these aspects should be carefully taken into account in order to correctly understand the intraoperative US exam.

4.3.2.2 Ultrasound Surgical Anatomy

Each neurosurgical approach leads to the exposure of specific area and structures. IOUS visualization varies accordingly to the approach and has never been standardized. Here we analyze the IOUS imaging obtained during the most common neurosurgical approaches, highlighting major anatomical landmarks for each approach as seen in IOUS along the two main plane of insonation (Figs. 4.6, 4.7, 4.8, 4.9, and 4.10).

In every panel the two main IOUS planes are displayed, along with the corresponding navigated MRI image and a three-dimensional model that explain the placement of the probe and the plane of insonation. Each approach of course can display only two planes of insonation, as it is not possible to obtain a plane that is perpendicular to the plane of the probe (Fig. 4.3).

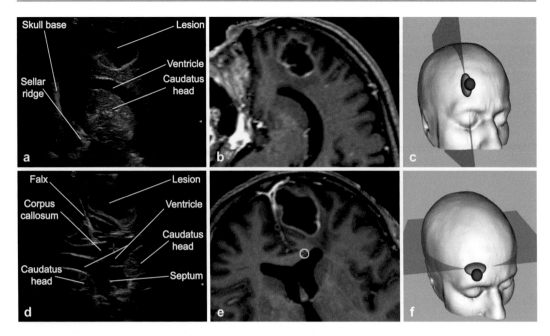

Fig. 4.6 Frontal approach. A case of a frontal-mesial metastasis is showed, which appears on IOUS as an hypoechoic cystic lesion surrounded by a bright hyperechoic rim. With the frontal approach, no coronal view is possible. (**a**, **b**) US and MR sagittal view, (**d**, **e**) US and MR axial view. (**c–f**) Three-dimensional model with probe positioning along the two main axes

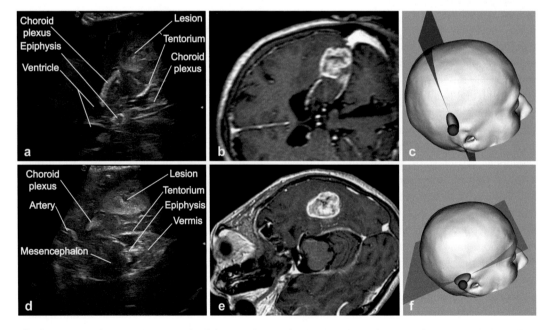

Fig. 4.7 Temporal approach. A case of a right posterior-temporal high-grade glioma is showed, which appears on IOUS as an hyperechoic lesion with calcifications and small cystic areas. With the temporal approach no sagittal view is possible. (**a**, **b**) US and MR coronal view, (**d**, **e**) US and MR axial view. (**c–f**) Three-dimensional model with probe positioning

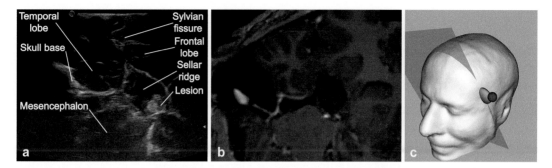

Fig. 4.8 Pterional approach. A case of a cystic cranio-pharyngioma is showed, which appears on IOUS as an hypoechoic cystic lesion with a nodular hyperechoic component surrounded by a bright hyperechoic rim. With the pterional approach, no sagittal view is possible. Furthermore in small pterional approaches, it is sometimes difficult to evaluate the axial plane. (**a**, **b**) US and MR semi-coronal view. (**c**) Three-dimensional model with probe positioning

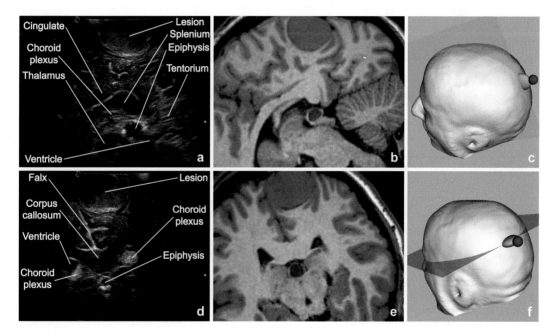

Fig. 4.9 Parietal approach. A case of a parasagittal meningioma, which appears on IOUS as an iso-hypoechoic homogenous lesion surrounded by a hyperechoic capsule. With the parietal approach no coronal view is possible. (**a**, **b**) US and MR sagittal view, (**d**, **e**) US and MR axial view. (**c**–**f**) Three-dimensional model with probe positioning

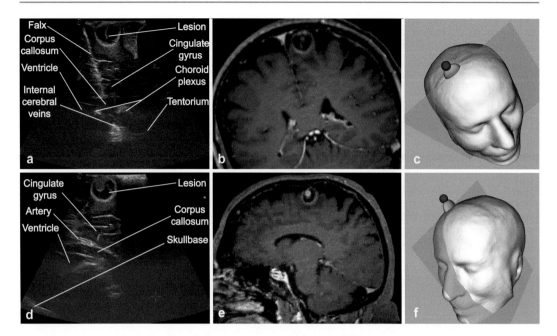

Fig. 4.10 Coronal approach. A case of a frontal-mesial lung metastasis is showed, which appears on IOUS as an hypoechoic cystic lesion with a nodular component surrounded by a bright hyperechoic rim. With the coronal approach, no axial view is possible. (**a, b**) US and MR coronal view, (**d, e**) US and MR sagittal view. (**c–f**) Three-dimensional model with probe positioning

References

1. Dorward NL, Alberti O, Velani B, Gerritsen FA, Harkness WF, Kitchen ND, Thomas DG (1998) Postimaging brain distortion: magnitude, correlates, and impact on neuronavigation. J Neurosurg 88(4):656–662. doi:10.3171/jns.1998.88.4.0656

2. Nimsky C, Ganslandt O, Cerny S, Hastreiter P, Greiner G, Fahlbusch R (2000) Quantification of, visualization of, and compensation for brain shift using intraoperative magnetic resonance imaging. Neurosurgery 47(5):1070–1079; discussion 1079–1080

3. Orringer DA, Golby A, Jolesz F (2012) Neuronavigation in the surgical management of brain tumors: current and future trends. Expert Rev Med Devices 9(5):491–500. doi:10.1586/erd.12.42

4. Stieglitz LH, Fichtner J, Andres R, Schucht P, Krahenbuhl AK, Raabe A, Beck J (2013) The silent loss of neuronavigation accuracy: a systematic retrospective analysis of factors influencing the mismatch of frameless stereotactic systems in cranial neurosurgery. Neurosurgery 72(5):796–807. doi:10.1227/NEU.0b013e318287072d

5. Cornelius JF, Slotty PJ, Kamp MA, Schneiderhan T, Steiger HJ, El-Khatib M (2014) Impact of 5-aminolevulinic acid fluorescence-guided surgery on the extent of resection of meningiomas-with special regard to high-grade tumors. Photodiagnosis Photodyn Ther. doi:10.1016/j.pdpdt.2014.07.008

6. Soleman J, Fathi AR, Marbacher S, Fandino J (2013) The role of intraoperative magnetic resonance imaging in complex meningioma surgery. Magn Reson Imaging 31(6):923–929. doi:10.1016/j.mri.2012.12.005

7. Uhl E, Zausinger S, Morhard D, Heigl T, Scheder B, Rachinger W, Schichor C, Tonn JC (2009) Intraoperative computed tomography with integrated navigation system in a multidisciplinary operating suite. Neurosurgery 64(5 Suppl 2):231–239. doi:10.1227/01.neu.0000340785.51492.b5; discussion 239–240

8. Reid MH (1978) Ultrasonic visualization of a cervical cord cystic astrocytoma. AJR Am J Roentgenol 131(5):907–908. doi:10.2214/ajr.131.5.907

9. Chacko AG, Kumar NK, Chacko G, Athyal R, Rajshekhar V (2003) Intraoperative ultrasound in determining the extent of resection of parenchymal brain tumours – a comparative study with computed tomography and histopathology. Acta Neurochir 145(9):743–748. doi:10.1007/s00701-003-0009-2; discussion 748

10. Chandler WF, Rubin JM (1987) The application of ultrasound during brain surgery. World J Surg 11(5):558–569

11. Ivanov M, Wilkins S, Poeata I, Brodbelt A (2010) Intraoperative ultrasound in neurosurgery – a practical guide. Br J Neurosurg 24(5):510–517. doi:10.3109/02688697.2010.495165

12. Machi J, Sigel B, Jafar JJ, Menoni R, Beitler JC, Bernstein RA, Crowell RM, Ramos JR, Spigos DG (1984) Criteria for using imaging ultrasound dur-

ing brain and spinal cord surgery. J Ultrasound Med 3(4):155–161

13. McGirt MJ, Attenello FJ, Datoo G, Gathinji M, Atiba A, Weingart JD, Carson B, Jallo GI (2008) Intraoperative ultrasonography as a guide to patient selection for duraplasty after suboccipital decompression in children with Chiari malformation Type I. J Neurosurg Pediatr 2(1):52–57. doi:10.3171/ped/2008/2/7/052

14. Rubin JM, Chandler WF (1987) The use of ultrasound during spinal cord surgery. World J Surg 11(5):570–578

15. van Velthoven V (2003) Intraoperative ultrasound imaging: comparison of pathomorphological findings in US versus CT, MRI and intraoperative findings. Acta Neurochir Suppl 85:95–99

16. Makuuchi M, Torzilli G, Machi J (1998) History of intraoperative ultrasound. Ultrasound Med Biol 24(9):1229–1242

17. Dohrmann GJ, Rubin JM (2001) History of intraoperative ultrasound in neurosurgery. Neurosurg Clin N Am 12(1):155–166, ix

18. Moiyadi A (2014) Objective assessment of intraoperative ultrasound in brain tumors. Acta Neurochir 156(4):703–704. doi:10.1007/s00701-014-2010-3

19. Prada F, Del Bene M, Moiraghi A, et al. (2015) From Grey Scale B-Mode to Elastosonography: Multimodal Ultrasound Imaging in Meningioma Surgery—Pictorial Essay and Literature Review, BioMed Research International, vol. 2015, Article ID 925729, 13 pages, 2015. doi:10.1155/2015/925729

20. Sosna J, Barth MM, Kruskal JB, Kane RA (2005) Intraoperative sonography for neurosurgery. J Ultrasound Med 24(12):1671–1682

21. Rygh OM, Selbekk T, Torp SH, Lydersen S, Hernes TA, Unsgaard G (2008) Comparison of navigated 3D ultrasound findings with histopathology in subsequent phases of glioblastoma resection. Acta Neurochir 150(10):1033–1041. doi:10.1007/s00701-008-0017-3; discussion 1042

Intraoperative Findings in Brain Tumor Surgery

Jan Coburger and Ralph W. König

5.1 Introduction

Intraoperative ultrasound for brain tumor surgery is an established technique in clinical routine. Application is noninvasive and cheap and can be applied repetitively during any stage of surgery without any harm for the patient [1]. Since the first description of intraoperative ultrasound (iUS) for neurosurgical use in 1982 by Chandler et al. [2], it has mainly been used for brain tumor surgery. Especially when approaching invasive intraaxial lesions, classical landmarks are often missing. iUS allows for a good orientation in these situations. Additionally, brain shift might change the anatomy significantly. Until introduction of intraoperative MRI (iMRI), iUS was the only means of intraoperative imaging depicting residual tumor during surgery [3]. Since its first use in neurosurgery until present, imaging capability has improved significantly. Dedicated probes for dedicated indications are available. Another important innovation is the integration of ultrasound devices into neuronavigation systems [4, 5]. By this method, iUS images can be referenced to a preoperative MRI dataset, which is displayed in the reconstructed plane of the 2D ultrasound image. Thus, interpretation of ultrasound findings becomes much easier and occurring brain shift can be identified early by comparing landmarks between intra and preoperative images. The main challenge when using iUS is interpretation of imaging findings. Especially during the course of surgery, artifacts might increase and identification of residual tumor can get challenging.

In the actual chapter, we will elucidate indications, techniques, and devices to optimize image quality in ultrasound-assisted brain tumor surgery.

5.2 Indications

As far as our experience goes, there is an indication for the use of ultrasound in every intraaxial brain tumor surgery. Each surgical step has its typical applications. At first, before incision of the dura, ultrasound helps to assess whether the target lesion is centered in the craniotomy (Fig. 5.1). Thus a simple verification of neuronavigation can be performed, and if needed, based on iUS findings, a safe extension of craniotomy can be performed before dural opening. Second, after dural opening by release of CSF or brain swelling, a significant brain shift may occur which unexpectedly changes surgical anatomy. At this step of surgery, a quick ultrasound sweep might help to identify the targeted lesion and important landmarks close by (Fig. 5.2). Further, the ultrasound

J. Coburger (✉) • R.W. König
Department of Neurosurgery, University of Ulm, Ludwig-Heilmeyerstr. 3, 89312 Günzburg, Germany
e-mail: Jan.coburger@uniklinik-ulm.de;
ralph.koenig@uni-ulm.de

© Springer International Publishing Switzerland 2016
F. Prada et al. (eds.), *Intraoperative Ultrasound (IOUS) in Neurosurgery: From Standard B-mode to Elastosonography*, DOI 10.1007/978-3-319-25268-1_5

provides information which gyrus is infiltrated and which might be spared. Since intraoperative ultrasound provides real-time information, when in doubt iUS provides more reliable information compared to neuronavigation.

In case of marked brain swelling due to large tumors with cystic components, intraoperative sonography allows for save inline cyst puncture or even ventricular puncture before removal of the solid tumor mass. By this means, a lot of tension is relieved which eases further dissection. If a deep-seated lesion is approached, an ultrasound-based planning of a trajectory is recommended for first, not missing the lesion. Second, the appropriate sulcus leading to a lesion can be verified (Fig. 5.3). During the course of surgery, we recommend using the ultrasound probe from time to time to adapt to surgically induced changes of the

Fig. 5.1 Typical application of intraoperative ultrasound before dural opening: assessment of craniotomy size with regard to the targeted lesion

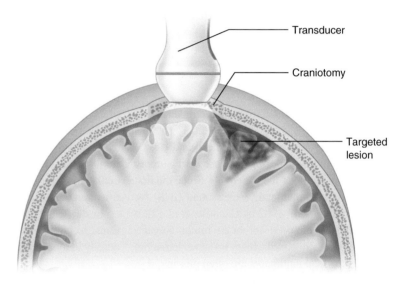

Fig. 5.2 Intraoperative screenshot of the neuronavigation system with an integrated 15 Mhz linear array transducer. The probes is at a coronary position depicting the border of an anaplastic astrocytoma between superior and medial temporal gyrus, right after dural opening before beginning of tumor resection. In the neuronavigation system, the tar-

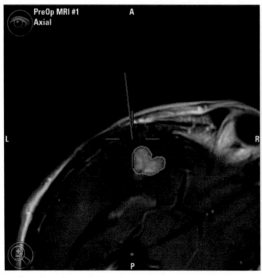
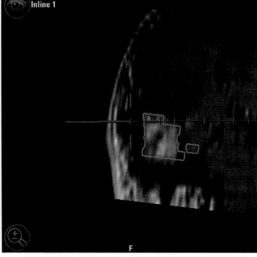

geted lesion is depicted with a *white line*. The *white arrows* show the direction of the occuring brain shift. Due to brainswelling the tumor is pushed in the direction of the ultrasound probe while it appears deeper in the corresponding MRI image of the neuronavigation

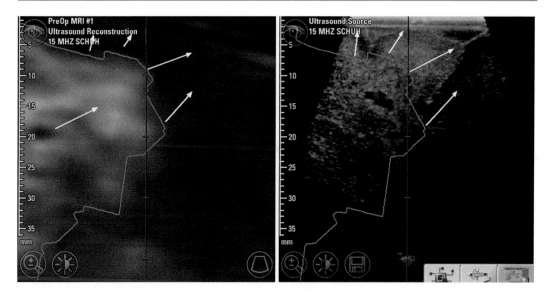

Fig. 5.2 (continued)

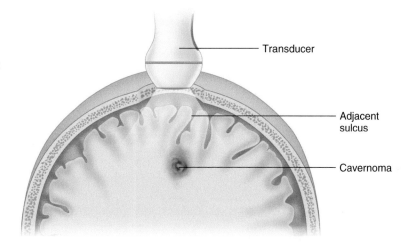

Fig. 5.3 Illustration of a small subcortical lesion (cavernoma). Ultrasound helps to find the best trajectory to the lesion. Even identification of an appropriate sulcus for a transsulcal approach can be performed

tumor or brain surface. Thus, it is easier to distinguish artifacts from residual tumor at a later stage of surgery (Fig. 5.4). Additionally adjacent structures like corpus callosum or the ventricles can be identified and the remaining distance tracked (Fig. 5.5). The short time consumed by the use of the iUS during tumor resection is easily outweighed by the increase of speed after gaining a confident idea of the surrounding structures.

Despite intraoperative orientation, the main indication for iUS while approaching intraaxial lesion is residual tumor assessment. Especially in low-grade glioma surgery, distinguishing between most likely tumor-free tissue and invasive glioma areas is challenging. Extent of resection is a significant predictor of overall survival in low- as well as high-grade gliomas [6, 7]. Intraoperative ultrasound helps to increase extent of resection [8]. Most contemporary iUS probes for intracranial use can discriminate between tumor and normal brain tissue at least at the beginning of surgery. In the chapter "tumor depiction," we will elucidate visibility of intra-axial tumors in more detail. An issue while performing iUS for residual tumor control is the appearance of surgery-induced artifacts which

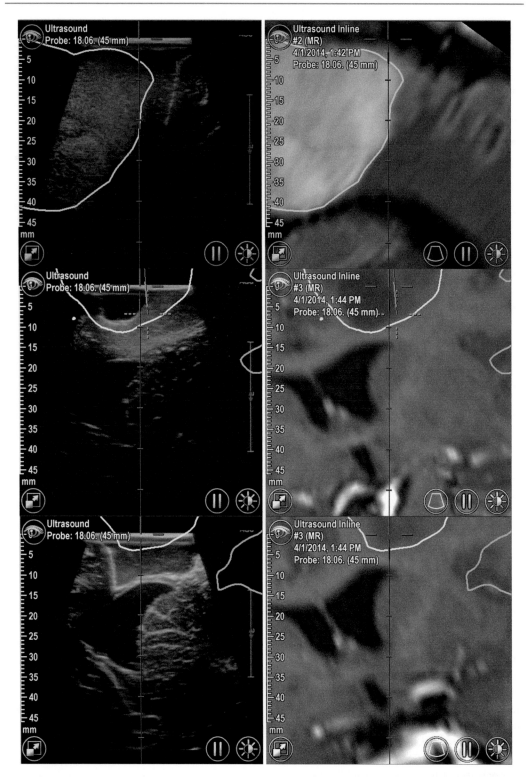

Fig. 5.4 Chronological screenshots of the neuronavigation system using linear array intraoperative ultrasound as a resection control. (1) Precise localization of the affected gyrus (*upper row*). (2) Identification of residual tumor and its adjacent anatomical structures (*middle row*). (3) Final inspection after tumor removal (*lower row*) (Copyright Coburger Acta neurochiru. 2015. Springer)

Fig. 5.5 Illustration of the important use of intraoperative US during resection. Continuously extent of resection and the distance to eloquent structures can be evaluated by this means

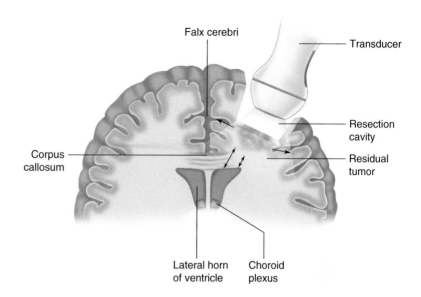

Falx cerebri

Transducer

Resection cavity

Residual tumor

Corpus callosum

Lateral horn of ventricle

Choroid plexus

lead to a lower specificity of iUS during the course of surgery [9]. Surgeons should be aware of possible false-positive findings due to blood or local brain contusions. We will discuss the different types of artifacts and options for image optimization later on in this chapter.

When using iUS referenced to a neuronavigation device, some systems provide the option for intraoperative 3D dataset acquisition. This allows to acquire a new intraoperative image set as a base for neuronavigation comparable to an intraoperative MRI Scan. We will comment on the topic of navigated iUS later on during this chapter.

5.3 Ultrasound Transducers for Intracranial Use

Ultrasound transducers for intracranial use need to have a small aperture to be positioned in typical craniotomies. Basically, there are 3 types of ultrasound transducers. Naming is based on the positioning of the piezoelectric crystals in the tip of the probes (Fig. 5.6).

Linear array transducers are producing parallel ultrasonic waves, thus creating a rectangular image with high-resolution and little artifacts. Based on the parallel sound waves, broadness of image is

limited by the aperture of the transducer. Therefore overview is limited in probes with a small footprint which are needed for intracranial use. Usually high frequencies are used for linear transducers leading to a high image resolution. However, there is an inverse correlation of penetration depth and increasing frequency. Typical frequencies used are 7–15 Mhz allowing for a penetration depth roughly from 2 to 7 cm. These parameters are highly variable based on tissue and transducer used.

Sector array transducers provide a triangular image leading to an increasing field of view and due to lower ultrasound frequencies increasing penetration depth. Typical frequencies are 4–8 Mhz. A sector array transducer has a small footprint; therefore it can be used even in small craniotomies or burr holes while still providing a useful overview of the tissue beneath [10]. Apparently, resolution is lower as in linear array transducers. Especially, increasing penetration depth is going along with decreased lateral resolution as the ultrasound waves are diverging. Matrix array transducers are a special type of sector array transducers with piezoelectric elements arranged like a chessboard. Thus, a real-time 3D image or live cross-plane visualization can be created. This increases overview and enhances understanding of the respective intracranial pathology [11].

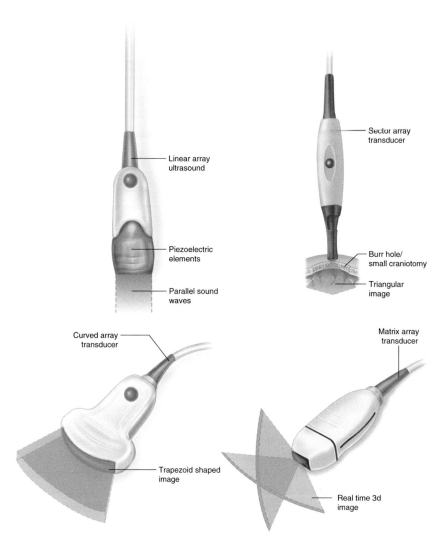

Fig. 5.6 The illustration shows the most commonly used types of transducers: (*left to right*) A linear array transducer produces parallel sound waves. Thus, resolution theoretically stays the same independent from depth. However the higher frequency leads to a decreased penetration depth. Sector array transducers have a small aperture and provide a trapezoid image. Therefore resolution is high close to the transducer and gets lower with increasing depth; however field of view is enlarged in the same matter. Thus, it allows for a wide field of view through small openings. A curved array transducer has a curved arrangement of the piezoelectric elements. It combines the previous transducer types. Penetration depth and field of view are increased while the field of view and the resolution close to the probe are still acceptable. Matrix array transducers are a special type of sector array transducers with piezoelectric elements arranged like on a chessboard. Thus, a real-time 3D image can be created

Curved array transducers are using lower frequencies between 2 and 10 Mhz. The positioning of the piezoelectric elements provides a compromise between the both types mentioned above. Curved array ultrasound was developed for abdominal ultrasound in order to provide a good resolution for superficial liver ultrasound as well as deep lesions. Therefore in the past probes were rather large. With recent technical advances, smaller probes for intracranial use became avail-

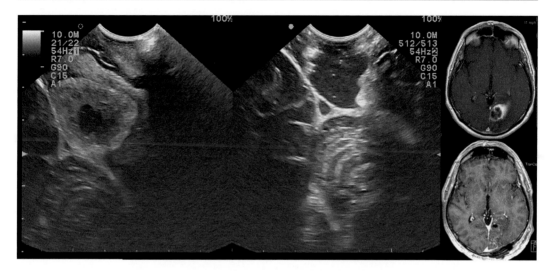

Fig. 5.7 Tangential iUS image of a supratentorial metastasis close to the falx using a curved array transducer. Tumor depiction after dural opening before start of tumor preparation (*left*). Final scan after tumor removal (*right*). Typical signals of residual blood at the floor of the resection cavity and along the tentorium. Residual tumor can only be excluded when comparing with previous images (no tumor along the tentorium). In comparison to the left image, a typical attenuation artifact is seen: The echo intensity of the cerebellar folia is increased (Images were provided by Mrs Nadji-Ohl, Department of Neurosurgery, Klinikum Stuttgart, Germany)

able, too. While resolution close to the transducer is high, it still provides a good overview due to the trapezoid imaging shape. Additionally, a penetration depth which allows for a good intracranial overview is provided (Fig. 5.7).

Depending on the indication several types of transducers may be required. Based on the technical features, the best compromise for typical intraaxial lesions is a small curved array transducer. For intraoperative use, hockey stick shaped linear array high-frequency transducer have been developed by several companies. The hockey stick shape allows for an intracavital use. Thus, penetration depth is not a limiting factor and the advantage of the high local resolution can be seized [12] (Fig. 5.8). In low- and high-grade glioma surgery, accuracy of residual tumor detection has been shown to be significantly higher as compared to conventional sector array probes [13, 14].

All types of ultrasound transducers can be referenced to a conventional neuronavigation system (Brainlab Vector vision, Brainlab AG, Feldkirchen, Germany) [15–17] or are available for the SonoWand system (Trondheim, Norway) as a dedicated device of navigated intraoperative ultrasound [3].

5.4   Tumor Depiction

Echogenicity of an intracranial tumor is dependent on cell density. With increased cell density especially in high-grade gliomas or in metastasis, a strong hyperechogenic signal can be depicted. Therefore, in low-grade gliomas, differentiation of the border of the lesion again might be more challenging. This effect is more pronounced in sector or curved array transducers as in linear array probes (Fig. 5.9). As a first step, we recommend to optimize contrast between most likely tumor-free tissue and tumor even before dural opening. Thus, based on imaging settings and depth of the lesion contrast, focus and other imaging settings can be optimized before any artifacts will obscure vision. In general contrast between "uninfiltrated" brain tissue and tumor is higher when using a linear array transducer [18]. Using a high-resolution linear array device, normal

Fig. 5.8 Typical application of a hockey stick-shaped linear array high-frequency transducer. Using the device, even small resection cavities can be scanned meticulously without use of a coupling fluid. Due to the small distance to the target and the absence of substances with different attenuation coefficients, attenuation artifacts are not relevant in this setup

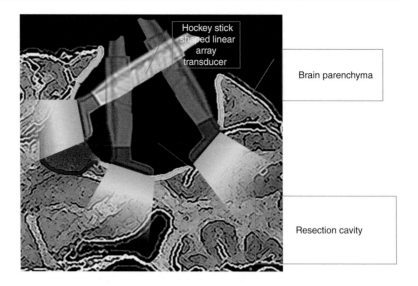

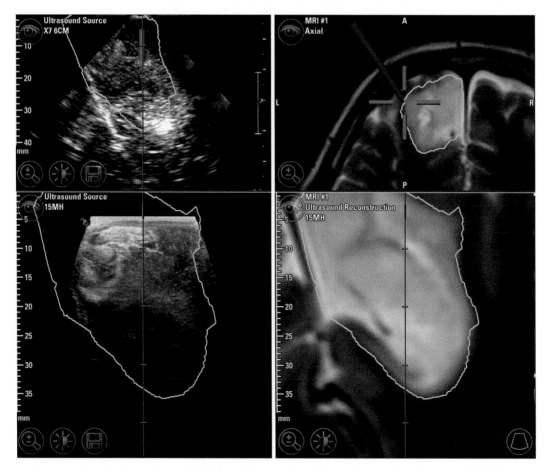

Fig. 5.9 Comparison of a transcortical image of navigated sector array intraoperative ultrasound (*upper row*) and linear array intraoperative ultrasound (*lower row*) with the corresponding iMRI image (T2 space) as calculated by the neuronavigation system (Copyright Coburger 2015 Acta Springer)

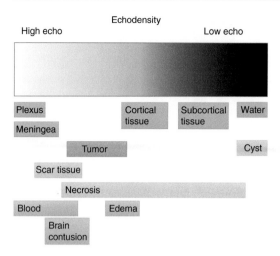

Fig. 5.10 Schematic illustration comparing signal intensity of typical anatomical structures (*green*), pathological structures (*red and yellow*), and surgically induced artifacts (*gray*)

subcortical tissue reflects very little signal and appears blackish. In Fig. 5.10 we provide a schematic table comparing signal intensity of typical anatomical structures (green), pathological structures (red and yellow), and surgically induced artifacts (gray). Obviously based on ultrasound conditions and transducers applied, a high variability may occur. Therefore, the provided gray scales have to be used as a schematic illustration and not as a calibration scale. Mair et al. established a grading system for ultrasound visibility of typical intracranial lesions and its discrimination at the border [19]. Grade 0 describes lesions that are not visible. Grade 1 describes tumors difficult to visualize without an exact border with normal brain tissue. Grade 2 is a clearly identifiable lesion lacking a clear boarder with normal brain tissue and grade 3 is a lesion clearly identifiable with a clear border with normal tissue. Figure 5.11 shows an illustration by the abovementioned authors describing grade I to grade III lesions. Figure 5.12 shows a characteristic of typical intracranial lesions by the same authors and the respective visibility using intraoperative ultrasound. The specific value of the cited study is that the authors used sector and linear array probes from 5 to 12 MHz. Therefore the data

provide an extraordinary overview on ultrasound depiction in 105 intracranial lesions. Depiction of tumor borders is not only dependent on the quality of the ultrasound images but on the type of lesion itself. Especially diffuse low-grade gliomas and lymphomas do not have a histologically defined border. In high-grade gliomas, intraoperative ultrasound is capable to identify different multiforme compartments of the solid lesion (Fig. 5.13) like necrosis, cysts, bleedings, irregular dense tumor, and the invasion zone. Especially the latter is difficult to differentiate from edema. A direct comparison of intraoperative MRI and sector and linear array ultrasound showed that linear array ultrasound is more sensitive for tumor detection than the other two techniques. However, it also detects the infiltration zone of the lesions (Table 5.1 unpublished data by our group). Histologically in glioblastoma, 60–100 % of tumor cell density can be found between 6 and 14 mm distant to the border of contrast enhancement [20]. Thus, an "over detection" might be favored by the surgeon. However, caution must be paid close to eloquent areas: Even though Gd-DTPA contrast enhancement does not enter an eloquent area, it does not mean the tumor does. New motor or language deficits are not only associated with decreased quality of life but with significant decreased overall survival [21]. Thus, when using these very detailed and sensitive imaging techniques in eloquent areas, we recommend using intraoperative monitoring. Additionally, surgeons should always keep in mind that contrast enhancement in iMRI and tumor depiction using intraoperative ultrasound might not be congruent at the border of the lesion. From our experience especially in low-grade gliomas, the signal of the FLAIR sequence of iMRI matches very well with iUS. In these entities, when using the iUS referenced to the navigation system, we recommend performing a T2 space sequence providing a 3D dataset with isovoxel for a precise reconstruction of the corresponding pre- or intraoperative MRI image (Fig. 5.14) In HGG, the same goes for a T1 MPRAGE with contrast.

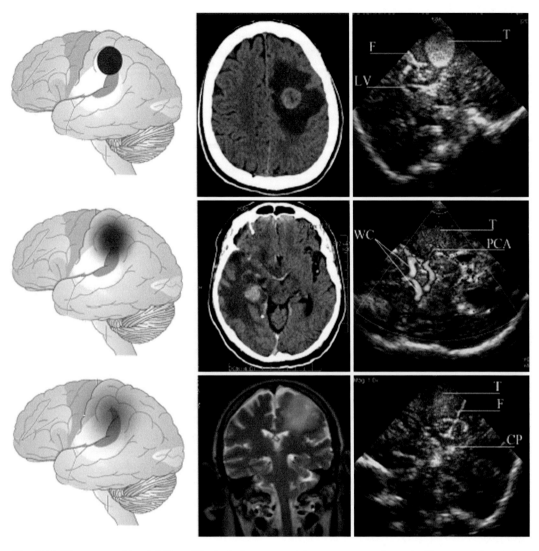

Fig. 5.11 Ultrasonographic visibility of brain lesions. (a) Grade III: the lesion is clearly identifiable and has a clear border with normal tissue; artistic representation, preoperative CT with contrast, and intraoperative ultrasound; coronal image. *T* tumor, *F* falx, *LV* lateral ventricles. (b) The lesion is clearly identifiable but has no clear border with normal tissue; CT with contrast—mesial temporal tumor, power angio mode. Tumor and its relationship to neighboring vessels are visible. *T* tumor, *WC* Willis circle, *PCA* posterior cerebral artery. (c) The lesion is difficult to visualize and has no clear border with normal tissue but remains identifiable on MRI (T2). *T* tumor, *F* falx, *CP* choroid plexus in the lateral ventricles (Copyright Springer Mair et al. Acta neuro 2013)

During resection, even though there is still solid tumor depicted under the microscope, we recommend periodic quick iUS sweeps to identify remaining tumor. This approach allows continuous assessment of subtle changes in ultrasound depiction between the solid tumor and the infiltration zone. Otherwise interpretation might be difficult at a later stage of sur-gery, when the solid tumor mass is almost removed.

Brain metastases are usually well circumscribed and have a defined border in MRI and in the corresponding ultrasound images. A typical depiction of a metastatic lesion is found in Fig. 5.7. Many mainly solid and circumscribed metastatic lesions show infiltrative zones, too. Usually in this

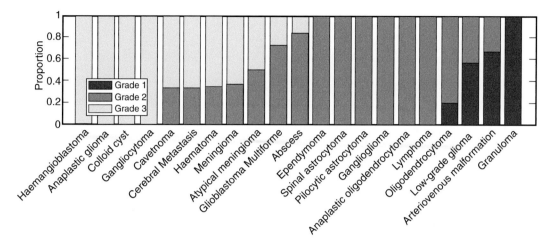

Fig. 5.12 Characterization of individual lesions using the grading system by Mair et al.: grade 0 describes lesions that are not visible. Grade 1 describes lesions difficult to visualize and no clear boarder with normal tissue. Grade 2 is a clearly identifiable lesion but no clear boarder with normal tissue and grade 3 is a lesion clearly identifiable with a clear boarder with normal tissue

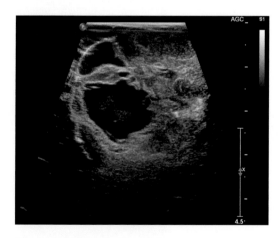

Fig. 5.13 High-resolution linear array ultrasound of a glioblastoma before tumor resection showing a precise differentiation of the "multiforme" parts of the lesion including necrosis and diffuse infiltration of the adjacent cortex

type of lesions, infiltration zones are found only in certain parts of the lesion (Fig. 5.15).

5.5 Artifacts and Image Optimization

When performing intracranial ultrasound, a good knowledge of typical ultrasound artifacts is crucial in order to interpret imaging results properly.

Type and extent of artifacts change from type of transducer used and based on the tissue assessed.

Therefore, a change of transducer during surgery might lead to a change of artifacts encountered.

Reverberation artifacts are reflections of ultrasound waves causing a mirrored image or multiple mirrored objects. In brain tumor surgery, this type of artifact might occur when visualizing a resection cavity filled with irrigation. The mirrored images will move when the transducer is changed. Thus, these artifacts are easily identifiable in most cases. Figure 5.16 shows a reverberation artifact as a combination of reflection at the resection cavity and the frontal skull base. Due to the level of artifacts, it is not possible to assess residual tumor in the presented position of the transducer.

Distortions and phase range artifacts are less common in neurosurgery since the brain is a rather homogenous organ. Usually this type of artifacts is elicited when a change of speed of sound occurs. Speed of sound in water, for example, is much higher as in brain tissue. Potential issues might be a resection cavity filled with fluid, a cystic lesion, or the ventricle. Errors in deep range might occur in this case since sound travels faster in water as in brain tissue. Thus

Table 5.1 Comparison of imaging results and histopathological diagnosis between intraoperative ultrasound and intraoperative MRI (check PowerPoint file Table for better visualization with histo-images)

Diagnosis of specimen	Intraoperative MRT			Sector array transducer (7.5 MHz)			Linear array transducer (15 MHz)		
	Negative	Intermediate	Positive	Negative	Intermediate	Positive	Negative	Intermediate	Positive
Tumor	26	17	27	26	3	12	8	3	32
Invasion zone	26	5	14	19	2	2	6	2	17
No tumor	1	0	0	1	0	0	1	0	0

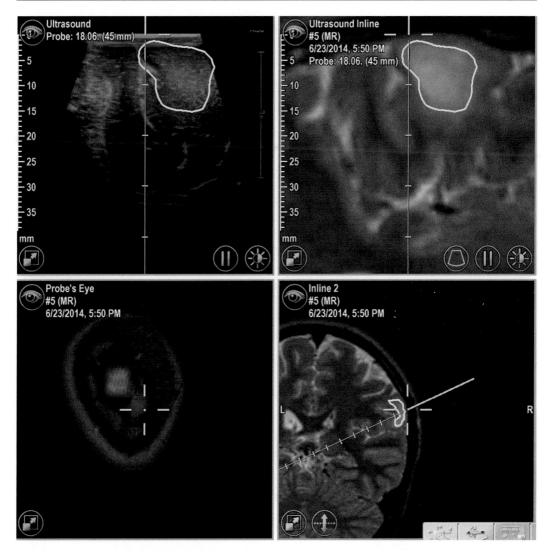

Fig. 5.14 Diffuse astrocytoma of the right operculum (*white line*). Linear array ultrasound (*left upper row*), corresponding T2 SPACE MRI in the neuronavigation

lesions behind a water-filled cavity could appear closer compared to lesions in brain tissue in the same depth.

A similar problem occurs based on different attenuations between different tissues. Attenuation in brain tissue is relatively high. Brain tissue even when infiltrated by a tumor is relatively homogenous with regard to attenuation. This is the reason for the high image quality in intraoperative ultrasound at the beginning of tumor resection. Water compared to brain tissue shows very little attenuation. Thus, if a resection

cavity is filled with irrigation, a significant difference in attenuation between brain tissue at the walls of the resection cavity and the bottom of the resection cavity is found. Therefore, a different signal at the floor of the cavity might be cause by this type of artifact (Fig. 5.7). This area might appear hyperechogenic and might be confound with residual tumor. Additionally, blood and micro-contusions may cause hyperechogenic signals. Therefore the importance of regular ultrasound sweeps during the process of tumor resection cannot be stressed enough. Thus, atten-

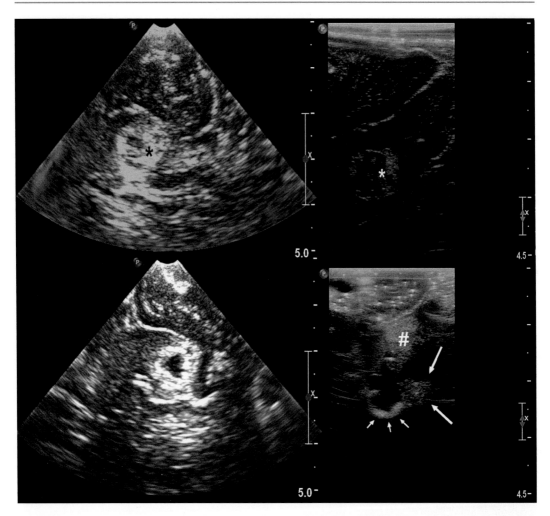

Fig. 5.15 *Upper row*: ultrasound images (US) of a deep-seated small metastasis (*) after dural opening before resection. Left 7 MHz US; right 15Mhz high-resolution US. *Lower row*: US of the resection cavity after microsurgical complete removal; left 7 Mhz US displays resection cavity with an adjacent sulcus due to a manipulation artifact; the tissue surrounding the resection cavity cannot be assessed. Right:15 Mhz high-resolution US reveals the infiltration zone of the metastasis (*big arrows*, histologically confirmed). Typical surgery-induced artifacts are shown: blood at the bottom of the resection cavity (*small arrows*) and a gelfoam (#) that was inserted

uation artifacts are easily identified since the artifact will move deeper and increase while the resection cavity is enlarged. We encourage also to take screenshots during this process in order to have images to compare to the actual ultrasound images (Fig. 5.17). Another option to decrease attenuation artifacts is to decrease distance of probe and object of interest. Most transducers for intracranial use can be inserted in typical resection cavities. Especially hockey stick shaped linear array high-frequency transducer facilitate intracavital use. Using such a device, irrigation is not needed in most cases (Fig. 5.8). In glioma surgery we found that intracavital use of hockey stick shaped linear array high-frequency transducer is feasible in over 90 % of cases [14]. Serra et al. described the approach to meticulously scan the whole resection cavity. This maneuver is best performed with a hockey stick-shaped probe at least in smaller resection cavities. The angle of the lateral wall is otherwise more difficult to assess. Additionally use of a linear array transducer is favorable for this approach since best tumor depiction is found close to the transducer.

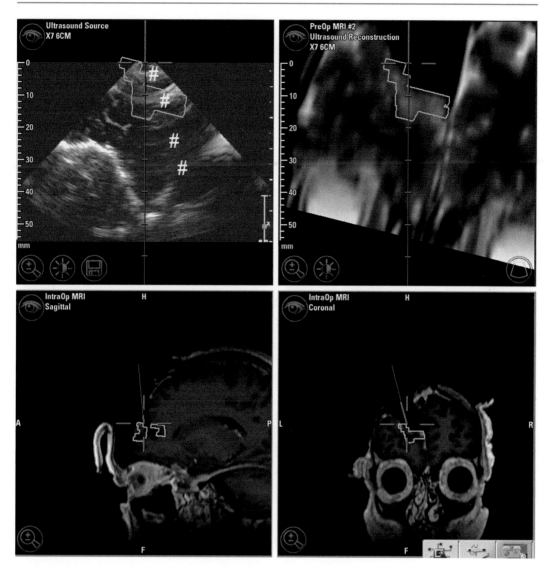

Fig. 5.16 Sector array ultrasound image (*upper left*) of a residual tumor of a diffuse astrocytoma confirmed by intraoperative MRI. Reconstructed intraoperative T2 according to the ultrasound position (*upper right*), sagittal T1+contrast (*lower left*), coronary T1+contrast (*lower right*); residual tumor is marked with a continuous *gray line*; reverberation artifacts are marked with #

A drawback of intracavital ultrasound using a transducer with a small footprint is the relatively small field of view and the uncommon perspective of the acquired images. Thus, orientation and retrieval of detected residual tumor can be challenging. A navigated use of the ultrasound transducer facilitates tumor detection. Additionally, a 3D sweep can be performed to get an "off-line" overview of the walls of the resection cavity (Fig. 5.17).

Another option to avoid attenuation artifacts easily feasible also with larger transducers is transcortical ultrasound. The lateral wall of the resection cavity is used as a "sound window" to assess the bottom and the walls for residual tumor (Fig. 5.18). Unsgaard et al. even propagated a second burr hole for continuous ultrasound imaging as a resection control in glioma surgery [22].

Selbek et al. described an acoustic coupling fluid with the same attenuation coefficient as

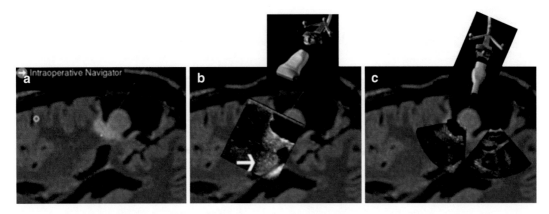

Fig. 5.17 Navigation display showing the reformatted ultrasound image slices on top of the corresponding reformatted MR image slice. Ultrasound image slice from 3D ultrasound volume acquired prior to start of resection (**a**), toward the end of resection with some tumor tissue remaining (**b**), and after completed tumor resection (**c**). Notice the signal enhancement below the cavity (marked with *arrows*) seen in c, which is not observed in a or b. Hence, it is very likely that the enhancement is an artifact and not remaining tumor (Selbek et al. [23] Acta Springer Copyright)

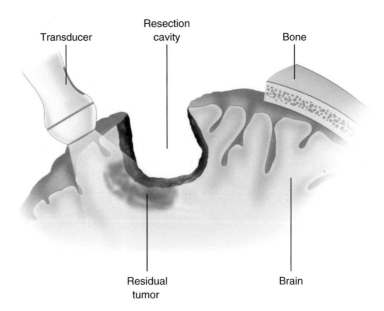

Fig. 5.18 Illustration of a tangential transcortical ultrasound in order to decrease attenuation artifacts

Transducer

Resection cavity

Bone

Residual tumor

Brain

brain tissue. Data are still preliminary. First results show a significantly better image quality compared to normal saline as irrigation fluid [23].

Irregularly shaped surfaces can be covered with an ultrasound gel pad to increase coupling of transducer and tissue. We frequently use these devices in peripheral nerve surgery at our center. In brain tumor surgery, it is rarely needed for this indication. However, gel pads can be useful to increase the distance between the tissue of interest and the probe. When using sector or some curved array transducer, a very superficial lesion might not be visualized appropriately due to the triangular or trapezoid field of view. Slightly increasing the distance with a gel pad might be enough to gain an adequate depiction.

Retrieval of areas of interest with the ultrasound which were found in the microscope and vice versa can be challenging. Orientation inside a resection cavity especially in deep lesions when visualization without retractor is not possible and neuronavigation for the ultrasound is not available adds to the problem. As a first step, anatomical landmarks which can be identified by both modalities like adjacent vessels, falx cerebri, ventricle, etc. should be identified. If this is not possible, artificial landmarks are a helpful option to "mark" certain areas of interest. Wong et al. described the use of a blood-soaked gelfoam as an internal fiducial [24]. Gelfoam is easily available and its intraoperative use is saved even if it remains in situ.

References

1. Wells PNT (1977) Ultrasonics in medicine and biology. Phys Med Biol 22(4):629
2. Chandler WF, Knake JE, McGillicuddy JE, Lillehei KO, Silver TM (1982) Intraoperative use of real-time ultrasonography in neurosurgery. J Neurosurg 57(2):157–163, Epub 1982/08/01. doi:10.3171/jns.1982.57.2.0157. PubMed
3. Unsgaard G, Gronningsaeter A, Ommedal S, Nagelhus Hernes TA (2002) Brain operations guided by real-time two-dimensional ultrasound: new possibilities as a result of improved image quality. Neurosurgery 51(2):402–411; discussion 11–12. Epub 2002/08/17. PubMed
4. Gronningsaeter A, Kleven A, Ommedal S, Aarseth TE, Lie T, Lindseth F et al (2000) SonoWand, an ultrasound-based neuronavigation system. Neurosurgery 47(6):1373–1379; discussion 9–80. PubMed
5. Schlaier JR, Warnat J, Dorenbeck U, Proescholdt M, Schebesch KM, Brawanski A (2004) Image fusion of MR images and real-time ultrasonography: evaluation of fusion accuracy combining two commercial instruments, a neuronavigation system and a ultrasound system. Acta Neurochir 146(3):271–277. doi:10.1007/s00701-003-0155-6
6. Sanai N, Berger MS (2008) Glioma extent of resection and its impact on patient outcome. Neurosurgery 62(4):753–764; discussion 264–266. Epub 2008/05/23. doi: 10.1227/01.neu.0000318159.21731.cf. PubMed
7. Smith JS, Chang EF, Lamborn KR, Chang SM, Prados MD, Cha S et al (2008) Role of extent of resection in the long-term outcome of low-grade hemispheric gliomas. J Clin Oncol 26(8):1338–1345, Epub 2008/03/08. doi:10.1200/jco.2007.13.9337. PubMed
8. Solheim O, Selbekk T, Jakola A, Unsgård G (2010) Ultrasound-guided operations in unselected high-grade gliomas—overall results, impact of image quality and patient selection. Acta Neurochir 152(11):1873–1886. doi:10.1007/s00701-010-0731-5
9. Gerganov VM, Samii A, Akbarian A, Stieglitz L, Samii M, Fahlbusch R (2009) Reliability of intraoperative high-resolution 2D ultrasound as an alternative

10. Masuzawa H, Kanazawa I, Kamitani H, Sato J (1985) Intraoperative ultrasonography through a burr-hole. Acta Neurochir 77(1–2):41–45. doi:10.1007/BF01402304
11. Bozinov O, Burkhardt JK (2012) Intra-operative computed-tomography-like real-time three-dimensional ultrasound in neurosurgery. World Neurosurg 78(1–2):5–7, Epub 2012/05/29. doi:10.1016/j.wneu.2012.05.025. PubMed
12. Serra C, Stauffer A, Actor B, Burkhardt JK, Ulrich NH, Bernays RL et al (2012) Intraoperative high frequency ultrasound in intracerebral high-grade tumors. Ultraschall Med 33(7):E306–E312, Epub 2012/11/07. doi:10.1055/s-0032-1325369. PubMed
13. Coburger J, Scheuerle A, Kapapa T, Engelke J, Thal DR, Wirtz CR et al (2015) Sensitivity and specificity of linear array intraoperative ultrasound in glioblastoma surgery: a comparative study with high field intraoperative MRI and conventional sector array ultrasound. Neurosurg Rev 38:499–509, Epub 2015/04/10. doi:10.1007/s10143-015-0627-1. PubMed
14. Coburger J, Scheuerle A, Thal DR, Engelke J, Hlavac M, Wirtz CR et al (2015) Linear array ultrasound in low-grade glioma surgery: histology-based assessment of accuracy in comparison to conventional intraoperative ultrasound and intraoperative MRI. Acta Neurochir (Wien) 157:195–206, Epub 2015/01/07. doi:10.1007/s00701-014-2314-3. PubMed
15. Coburger J, König RW, Scheuerle A, Engelke J, Hlavac M, Thal DR et al (2014) Navigated high frequency ultrasound: Description of technique and first clinical comparison with conventional intracranial ultrasound. World Neurosurg
16. Sure U, Benes L, Bozinov O, Woydt M, Tirakotai W, Bertalanffy H (2005) Intraoperative landmarking of vascular anatomy by integration of duplex and Doppler ultrasonography in image-guided surgery. Technical note. Surg Neurol 63(2):133–141; discussion 41–42. Epub 2005/02/01. doi:10.1016/j.surneu.2004.08.040. PubMed
17. Tirakotai W, Miller D, Heinze S, Benes L, Bertalanffy H, Sure U (2006) A novel platform for image-guided ultrasound. Neurosurgery 58(4):710–718; discussion −8. Epub 2006/04/01. doi: 10.1227/01. neu.0000204454.52414.7a. PubMed
18. Coburger J (2015) Linear array ultrasound: a dedicated tool for a dedicated application. Acta Neurochir (Wien) 157:959–960. doi:10.1007/s00701-015-2406-8, Epub 2015/04/08. PubMed
19. Mair R, Heald J, Poeata I, Ivanov M (2013) A practical grading system of ultrasonographic visibility for intracerebral lesions. Acta Neurochir 155(12):2293–2298. doi:10.1007/s00701-013-1868-9
20. Yamahara T, Numa Y, Oishi T, Kawaguchi T, Seno T, Asai A et al (2010) Morphological and flow cytometric analysis of cell infiltration in glioblastoma: a com-

parison of autopsy brain and neuroimaging. Brain
Tumor Pathol 27(2):81–87, PubMed

21. McGirt MJ, Mukherjee D, Chaichana KL, Than
KD, Weingart JD, Quinones-Hinojosa A (2009)
Association of surgically acquired motor and language
deficits on overall survival after resection of glioblastoma multiforme. Neurosurgery 65(3):463–469;
discussion 9–70. Epub 2009/08/19. doi:10.1227/01.
neu.0000349763.42238.e9. PubMed

22. Unsgaard GK (1999) Atle; ommedal, steinar; gronningsaeter, aage. An ultrasound-based neuronavigation system, a good solution to the brain-shift problem.
Neurosurgery 45(3):696

23. Selbekk T, Jakola AS, Solheim O, Johansen TF, Lindseth
F, Reinertsen I et al (2013) Ultrasound imaging in neurosurgery: approaches to minimize surgically induced
image artefacts for improved resection control. Acta
Neurochir (Wien) 155(6):973–980, Epub 2013/03/06.
doi:10.1007/s00701-013-1647-7.   PubMed   PMID:
23459867; PubMed Central PMCID: PMC3656245

24. Wong JM, Governale LS, Friedlander RM (2011) Use
of a simple internal fiducial as an adjunct to enhance
intraoperative ultrasound-assisted guidance: technical
note. Neurosurgery 69(1 Suppl Operative):ons34–
ons39;   discussion   ons9.   Epub   2011/02/25.
doi:10.1227/NEU.0b013e3182124851. PubMed

Intraoperative Findings in Spinal Lesions

Ignazio G. Vetrano and Francesco Prada

6.1 Introduction

Spinal tumor can arise from the spinal cord, nerve roots, vertebrae, meninges, or cauda equina. More than 2/3 of spinal tumors are non-malignant lesions. As far as their origin and relationship with neural structures is concerned, spinal tumors can be divided into extradural, intradural extra-medullary or intramedullary. Meningiomas, nerve sheath tumors, and ependymomas are the most frequent histotypes encountered [9, 40, 44]. Primary spinal cord tumors are one of the rarest types of tumors, representing about 4–8 % of all central nervous system tumors [9, 40].

Surgical excision represents the standard treatment option, although it still yields a considerable risk of neurological deficits. This is particularly true in surgical removal of intramedullary tumors, where a myelotomy must be performed [5, 17, 39, 44]. Five to forty percent of patients who undergo surgical resection of an intradural tumor can develop new neurological deficits [5, 39].

Recently, the introduction of new surgical tools, along with intraoperative electrophysiological monitoring, has contributed in significantly reducing the risks of postoperative neurological deficits [1, 6, 17, 39].

Intraoperative imaging tools for spinal tumor surgery could improve this aspect of surgery, reducing the manipulation of neural structures, which may lead to worsening of neurological symptoms.

Magnetic resonance imaging (MRI) represents the gold standard for diagnosis and assessment of intradural tumors. Nevertheless, MRI may not always accurately differentiate between intramedullary and extramedullary lesions. Furthermore, intraoperative MRI is not yet a standardized tool in spinal tumor surgery, harboring many technical limitations.

In recent years, the use of IOUS guidance has become progressively more widespread during neurosurgical procedures for brain tumor removal [2, 15, 19, 27, 30–32, 34].

However, US appearance of spinal tumors has been described in few studies until now, and the role of IOUS is not yet well standardized in this surgical field [2–4, 10, 12, 15, 19, 22, 24–26, 29, 33, 35–38, 42, 43, 46].

I.G. Vetrano, MD (✉)
Department of Neurosurgery, Fondazione IRCCS
Istituto Neurologico C. Besta,
Via G. Celoria 11, 20133 Milan, Italy

Università degli Studi di Milano, Milan, Italy
e-mail: ignazio.vetrano@unimi.it

F. Prada
Department of Neurosurgery, Fondazione IRCCS
Istituto Neurologico C. Besta,
Via G. Celoria 11, 20133 Milan, Italy
e-mail: francesco.prada@istituto-besta.it

© Springer International Publishing Switzerland 2016
F. Prada et al. (eds.), *Intraoperative Ultrasound (IOUS) in Neurosurgery:
From Standard B-mode to Elastosonography*, DOI 10.1007/978-3-319-25268-1_6

The first case of ultrasonographic visualization of a spinal tumor was reported in 1978 by Reid, who described a cervical spinal astrocytoma [36]. In 1984, Jokich presented a B-mode analysis of spinal cord alteration, focusing on spinal motion, in a limited series of neoplastic and degenerative disorders of the spine [18]. In 1991, Epstein presented a retrospective study about the characteristics on ultrasound of a very large series of intramedullary lesions [10]. Other studies regarded traumatic spinal column surgery [7, 14, 16, 24], syringomyelia [8], diastematomyelia [13], and degenerative vertebral disk disorders [16, 20, 21, 23, 28]. Obviously, some of these studies present some limitations due to technical characteristics of the machines available at the time. Regarding the surgery of spinal tumors, the application of IOUS has not been widely used thus far [4, 11, 12, 25, 26, 29, 33, 37]. More recently, Regelsberger reported a large series of 78 patients, in which IOUS was used to localize spinal tumors [35]. In 2012, Bozinov focused on the use of IOUS for localization and resection of intramedullary cavernomas [3]. A recent paper from Shamov attempted to assess the impact of IOUS on resection of extramedullary tumors [42]. The application of elastography on spinal cord intraoperative examination represents to date only a sporadic report [45].

All these studies tried to evaluate and validate the routine application of intraoperative ultrasound-guided surgery of spinal tumors.

6.2 Instruments and Technique

A variety of probes can be used for intraoperative imaging of the spine, but the localization of the surgical access site requires an end-fire configuration for the IOUS probes. For evaluating the spinal cord, very high frequencies of 10 MHz or greater can be effectively used and provide outstanding spatial and temporal resolution. At our institution, we routinely use a last-generation US device, also equipped with navigation system,(MyLab, Esaote, Italy) with a linear multifrequency (3–11 MHz) probe for deep-seated lesions or high frequency (7–18 MHz) for small or superficial lesions.

To achieve access to the spinal canal for tumor removal, patients are operated in prone position. The spinal region of interest is usually localized and marked with radiographic guidance before skin incision.

Standard hemilaminectomy, laminectomy, or laminotomy are performed. Patients are then examined with transdural and direct sonography. The probe is placed in a transparent plastic surgical sterile sheath (CIVCO, USA), filled with US-specific transducing gel, to guarantee acoustic coupling at the transducer membrane. The probe is then placed in the surgical cavity that is irrigated with saline solution. Differently than brain IOUS examinations, only two major planes of insonation (axial and sagittal axes) are allowed (Fig. 6.1). Standard B-mode imaging is acquired before dural opening, in order to check if the bone removal is sufficient and the lesion fully exposed. Furthermore, the lesion is identified and measured on the two axes. Tumor US characteristics, boundaries, and specific anatomical landmarks are acquired.

All lesions can be defined as hyperechoic, isoechoic, or hypoechoic as compared to the surrounding tissues. Other characteristics of the lesions that are taken into account are diffuse or circumscribed appearance, homogeneity versus heterogeneity, presence of calcifications, and/or cystic/necrotic areas as well as their relationships with the surrounding structures.

Transdural US examination is helpful in adapting the entity of surgical exposure to the actual measures of the lesions, visualizing precisely the craniocaudal and lateral extension of the tumor. Targeting bone removal before dural opening reduces the risk of direct injury of the exposed neural structures. This could also avoid venous bleeding inside the intradural compartment, due to decompressed epidural venous plexuses.

The use of color-mode Doppler US could be helpful in identifying major vessels surrounding lesions: in example, cervical tumor could sometimes displace vertebral arteries.

IOUS also allows the visualization of nerve rootlets and dentate ligaments, facilitating the mobilization of neural structures, especially in cases that have a predominant anterior location.

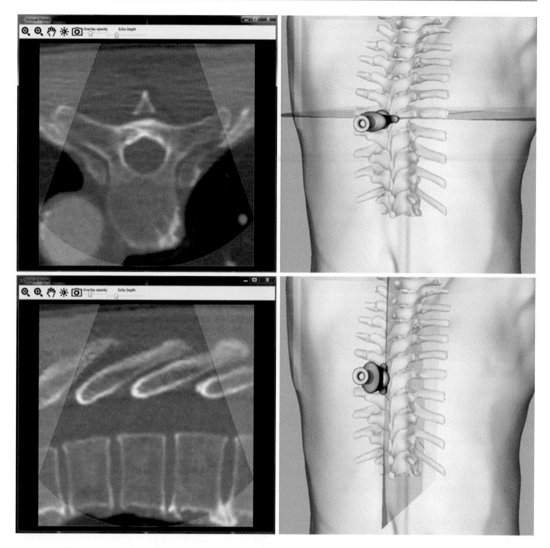

Fig. 6.1 US probe on a three-dimensional model and corresponding planes of insonation reconstructed from a CT. *Upper panel* shows an axial insonation plan, and *lower panel* shows a sagittal insonation plan

All intramedullary lesions are also evaluated with IOUS after dural opening, in order to correctly place the myelotomy and to adjust its length so to fully visualize and remove the lesion without unnecessary neural tissue manipulation.

Usually, the spinal cord appears enlarged due to the lesion which is partially or completely embedded within. In case of infiltrative lesions, the appearance is isoechoic to the spinal cord and the surface between tumor and myelin cannot be clearly distinguished. The surgical procedure should be limited to performing an internal decompression and obtaining a definitive histological diagnosis.

6.3   Limitations

A few technical limitations have to be considered: the size of the tip of the currently used US probe (1×3.5 cm) sometimes could be larger than the actual surgical field.

In case of diffuse bleeding or excessive use of hemostatic materials, which are highly hyperechoic [41], it is difficult to visualize the surrounding parenchyma.

The evaluation of neoplastic remnants could be a challenge for intramedullary tumors. In fact, perifocal edema hinders the accurate differentiation of medullar structures to residual pathological tissue.

The quality of triggered data always depends by the stability of the patient's heart rate, breath hold and probe position. Obviously, only examination on axial and sagittal axes is possible. The limited probe mobility also hinders the use of Doppler imaging, reducing the possibility to visualize vessels that run perpendicular to the insonation angle.

To date, the role of elastography is very limited in spinal cord tumor evaluation, differently from its application on brain tumors. In fact, external pressure onto neural structures that are already compromised is unacceptable. Further studies could be necessary to evaluate the role of this technique.

6.4   B-Mode Anatomical Landmarks

After bone removal, the spinal cord is visualized through the intact dura, which appears as a thin, linear, or curvilinear echogenic structure surrounding the dorsal and ventral portions of the cord. The spinal cord itself is quite homogeneous and hypoechoic. B-mode examination distinguishes the bright echogenic line or parallel double line of the central ependymal canal, which is located centrally inside the spinal cord. Alterations of the central canal represent an indi-

rect signal that could indicate the presence of intramedullary disease processes.

The cord is surrounded by hypoechoic cerebrospinal fluid within the subarachnoid spaces. The spinal cord is attached to the dural sac by the dentate ligaments, which appear as echogenic linear structures extending from the dura to the lateral margins of the cordon on each side. Nerve roots are also seen as linear echogenic structures within the subarachnoid space; these can be seen exiting along the ventral lateral surface of the sac and can also be visualized as a conglomerate group of linear echoes below the cord in the region of the cauda equina (Fig. 6.2).

The size and shape of the cord and sac vary by location. In fact, the thoracic cord is usually the thinnest and most spherical, while the cervical cord is somewhat thicker and somewhat more oval. Caudally, the thoracic cord tapers to end in the conus medullaris.

Vertebral bodies under the dural sac appear as hyperechoic structures, separated by hypoechoic intervertebral disks.

The spinal cord shows two different rhythmic movements, one synchronous with the heart beat and one with the respiratory acts [18]. Alteration of the pulsation of the spinal cord represents an indirect signal of the presence of a lesion.

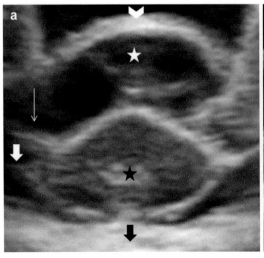
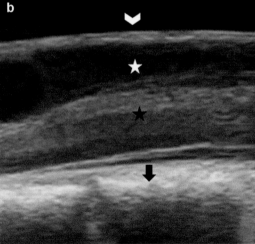

Fig. 6.2 IOUS axial (**a**) and sagittal (**b**) B-mode transdural imaging of spinal cord herniation. IOUS is able to identify the spinal cord (*black asterisk*) with its features as well as the surrounding structures: the dura mater (*arrow-*head), cerebrospinal fluid space (*star*), posterior rootlets (*thin arrow*), dentate ligament (*thick arrow*), and vertebral body (*black arrow*)

6.5 IOUS in Spinal Lesions

Spinal lesions visualized with IOUS imaging presents typical findings, related to the histopathology and location. IOUS findings for lesions affecting spinal compartment are summarized in Table 6.1. Hence are reported descriptions of ultrasonographic characteristics of the most frequent histotype for all compartments.

6.5.1 Extradural Tumors

Extradural lesions arise from bone and connective structures and include many osteal and soft tissue malignant tumors, but the most frequent extradural tumors admitted at neurosurgical centers are represented by nerve sheath schwannomas. This kind of lesion is usually completely visible after bone removal. The bone scalloping due to the slow growth of benign tumors allows room for a good visualization of the distal portion of the lesion. Such lesions appear well circumscribed, with a hyperechoic capsule and a hypoechoic homogeneous texture. In case of extradural tumors, the adjunct of Doppler examination represents an ulterior aid in clarifying the relationship between lesions and vascular structures.

6.5.2 Intradural Extramedullary Tumors

Extramedullary tumors include principally meningiomas and intradural schwannomas; other lesions, both benign and malignant, are represented by lipomas, dermoids, or metastases.

All of them can be easily recognized in B-mode because they appear more echogenic than myelinic structures. They are usually surrounded, at least in part, by subarachnoid fluid, making tumor margins quite visible. The spinal cord is often displaced and at times may appear reduced in caliber, but the central spinal canal will be maintained.

This is helpful in distinguishing an intramedullary from an extramedullary lesion.

Oscillations of the spinal cord before dural opening, due to cardiac pulsation and respiratory movements, may sometimes be diminished at the site of a highly compressive extramedullary mass. Paradoxically, if there is a great compression, transmitted pulsations from compressed spinal arteries may increase these oscillations.

6.5.2.1 Meningiomas

Spinal meningiomas are more common in the thoracic region with a female/male ratio of 10:1. Meningiomas appear as discrete, ovular, well-

Table 6.1 Ultrasonographic B-mode characteristics of spinal tumors

Histotype	B-mode features		
	Echogenicity	Appearance	Cystic-like areas and/or necrosis
Neurinoma	Often with low or isoechoic	Circumscribed	Sometimes microcystic or macrocystic appearance
Filum terminale ependymoma	Hyperechoic	Circumscribed	No
Meningioma	Hyperechoic	Circumscribed	Microcysts
Chordoma	Hypoechoic	Circumscribed	No
Metastasis	Variably hyperechoic	Nodular Heterogeneous	Large cysts/necrotic areas
Intramedullary ependymoma	Hyperechoic	Circumscribed Homogeneous	Small/microcysts, syrinx
Hemangioblastoma	Variably hyperechoic	Nodular Homogeneous	Perilesional cyst, macrocystic appearance
Cavernoma	Hyperechoic	Circumscribed	No
Glioma	Variably hyperechoic	Heterogeneous	Sometimes intralesional or perilesional cyst

circumscribed, mildly hyperechoic lesions, compared to normal spinal cord and cerebrospinal fluid, with a finely granular, homogeneous appearance for the presence of calcifications (Fig. 6.3). The dural attachment, in most cases, is not visible since it is anterolateral. The spinal cord and rootlets are visible and displaced to the opposite side.

6.5.2.2 Schwannomas

Intradural schwannomas present as ovular, circumscribed, mildly hyperechoic lesions, though less homogeneous as compared to meningiomas (due to the presence of some microcystic areas). In these lesions, the spinal cord is often displaced

anterolaterally and contralaterally, but in some cases, the nerve rootlets appeared stretched posterior to the lesion (Fig. 6.4).

The arachnoidal interface between the tumor and the spinal cord is usually intact and visible as a bright hyperechoic thin line, except for some cases such as large schwannomas or a melanotic schwannoma. This is due to disruption of the arachnoid plane by the tumor.

6.5.2.3 Filum Terminale Ependymomas

Ependymomas arising from cauda equina structures are quite different from intramedullary ones. On B-mode examination, they usually show a

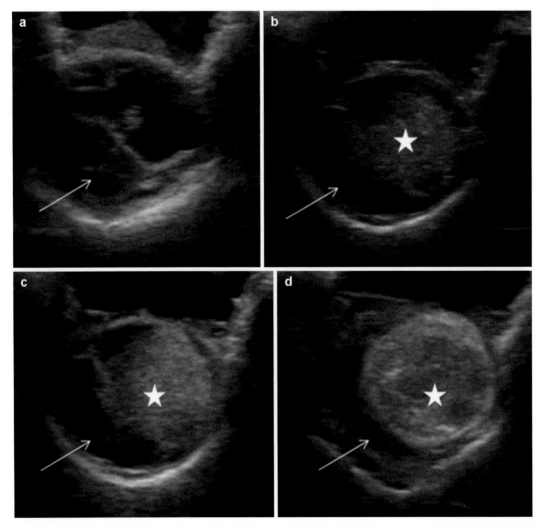

Fig. 6.3 Sequence showing axial (**a–d**) B-mode scans of a meningioma (*star*) that appears capsulated, homogeneous, and roundly shaped. The spinal cord is pushed anteriorly and laterally (*arrow*), with distortion of the arachnoidal structure (which is not recognizable due to the presence of the lesion)

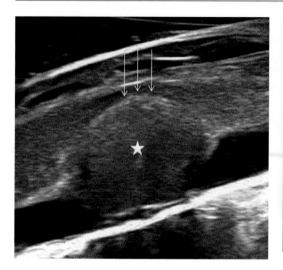

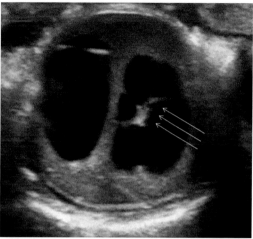

Fig. 6.4 Thoracic schwannoma: IOUS scan identifies the tumor (*star*) compressing the surrounding spinal cord, which appears slightly enlarged and hyperechoic due to spinal cord edema; tumor-myelinic structures interface is still identifiable (*triple arrows*)

Fig. 6.5 Syrinx or peritumoral cyst? In general, the septations within tumor-derived cysts are thicker and more nodular compared to the thin septations (*arrows*) that maybe seen with a syrinx, in case of intramedullary lesions

clear demarcation from the surrounding nerve tracts, with a homogeneous signal intensity: they usually are hyperechoic as compared to myelin. Usually no cystic areas or necrosis is present.

6.5.3   Intramedullary Tumors

Intramedullary tumors are usually distinguishable from their extramedullary counterparts. They usually appear variably hyperechoic when compared to the spinal cord, with a circumscribed and homogeneous aspect, sometimes with intralesional or perilesional cysts or dilation of the central ependymal canal. The spinal cord, if normal, usually appears hypoechoic and homogeneous. At times, it can appear as hyperechoic due to the presence of tissue edema; in these cases, it may be difficult to distinguish between the lesion and the surrounding compressed and/or infiltrated spinal cord.

Some intramedullary tumors such as hemangioblastoma or ependymomas have a typical appearance, including cystic intratumoral or peritumoral structures. These are expression of the inherent nature of the underlying tumor, whereas other times may represent areas of cystic degeneration within a solid tumor. Hemorrhagic

material or proteinaceous material may give a relatively hyperechoic appearance to these cystic tumors. However, tumor-related syrinx could also be present and be difficult to distinguish from peritumoral cysts. In general, the septations within tumor-derived cysts are thicker and more nodular compared to the thin septations that may be seen with a syrinx (Fig. 6.5).

Otherwise, intramedullary gliomas reflect, also sonographically, their histopathological characteristics. Due to their glial origin, it can be very difficult to distinguish them from medullary tissue.

If lesions are deeply embedded into the spinal cord and do not emerge on its surface, is necessary to perform a myelotomy along the posterior sagittal sulcus, which not always is clearly discernible. In these intramedullary cases, IOUS is used to correctly place the myelotomy, thus minimizing spinal cord manipulation. In other cases, for example, with gliomas, the tumor appears isoechoic to the spinal cord and the surface between tumor and myelin is not clearly recognized. The surgical procedure can be limited to performing an internal decompression and obtaining a specimen for histopathological examination; IOUS represents a guide for obtaining pathological tissue specimen.

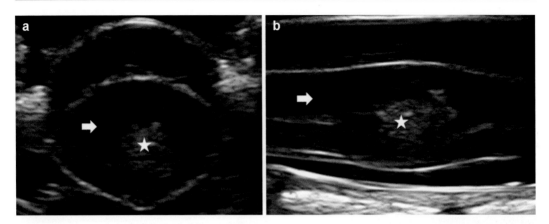

Fig. 6.6 Intramedullary ependymoma (*star*). Axial (**a**) and sagittal (**b**) IOUS findings show the enlarged spinal cord (*thick arrows*) without apparent cord edema. The central ependymal canal is also well demonstrated with IOUS

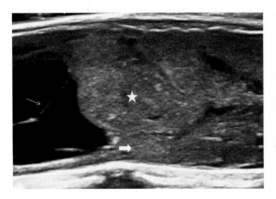

Fig. 6.7 Axial B-mode scan of a hemangioblastoma, depicting an ovalar lesion (*star*) surrounded by cystic cavity with septations (*thin arrow*). The spinal cord (*thick arrow*) appears quite hyperechogenic, due to the edema

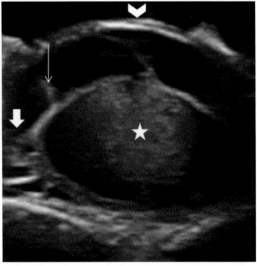

Fig. 6.8 Axial visualization of intramedullary cavernoma (*star*), embedded into the spinal cord that appears hypoechoic. Cavernomas usually have a highly hyperechoic presentation, with microcystic and microcalcification areas. Other structures are visible: the dura mater (*arrowhead*), posterior rootlets (*thin arrow*), and dentate ligament (*thick arrow*)

6.5.3.1 Ependymomas

Intramedullary ependymomas appear hyperechoic as compared to neural tissues, with a circumscribed homogeneous aspect. They are usually associated to some small/microcystic polar areas, sometimes to syrinx (Fig. 6.6).

6.5.3.2 Hemangioblastomas

Hemangioblastoma is a highly vascular intramedullary lesion that could also extend into the intradural space as well. It may be superficial while in other cases may present deeply embedded within the spinal cord. It appears hyperechoic with a nodular, homogeneous aspect, often with perilesional cyst and macrocystic appearance. An associated syrinx could be pres-

ent and difficult to distinguish from tumoral cysts (Fig. 6.7).

6.5.3.3 Cavernomas

Intramedullary cavernous malformations are very rare lesions. Cavernomas have a highly hyperechoic presentation, with microcystic and microcalcification areas (Fig. 6.8). They appear less circumscribed with respect to other intra-

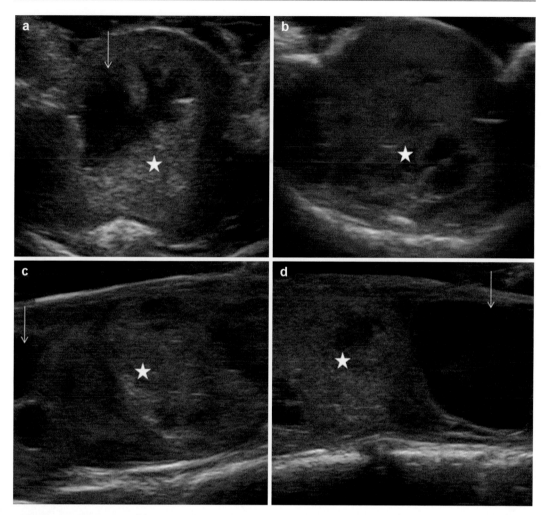

Fig. 6.9 Axial (**a**, **b**) and sagittal (**c**, **d**) scans of intramedullary low-grade astrocytoma (*star*). The lesion, highly infiltrative, appears with fine, granular hyperechogenicity and blurred margins. The border between intact myelin and tumor is not evident. The spinal cord is enlarged. Some intratumoral cysts are evident (*arrows*)

medullary lesions like hemangioblastoma. Cavernomas may be superficial, right on the surface of the spinal cord, and other times embedded into the spinal cord and covered by myelinic structures. It is at times possible to detect remnants of hemosiderin along the resection line, due to intralesional bleeding.

6.5.3.4 Astrocytomas

Astrocytomas are highly infiltrative and sometimes hypervascular tumors. Due to their origin from the glia, it can be very difficult to distinguish them from the surrounding spinal cord.

Usually, the border between intact myelin and tumor is not sonographically evident. The spinal cord appears enlarged. This kind of lesions usually appears with fine, granular hyperechogenicity and blurred margins. In such case, IOUS guides to obtain specimen for intraoperative histopathological examination (Fig. 6.9).

Conclusions

IOUS appears to be a fast, safe, and economic tool and represents a real-time dynamic procedure that can be performed during spinal tumor surgery.

This technique allows full evaluation of the lesion before dural opening and adds valuable real-time information in regard to the anatomic relationships between the tumor and the surrounding neural and vascular tissues.

IOUS also allows to tailor the extension of the neurosurgical approach to the true extent of the tumor. This avoids further bone removal while the dura is already opened with the edematous spinal cord protruding through the opening, thus avoiding possible surgical complications.

IOUS could be helpful in adapting and maybe reducing the extent of myelotomy in cases of intramedullary tumors, reducing unnecessary spinal cord manipulation.

The evaluation of the anatomy underneath the surface of the surgical field may improve the surgical strategy. This facilitates neural and vascular structure manipulation and ultimately the surgical removal of the lesion.

References

1. Avila EK, Elder JB, Singh P, Chen X, Bilsky MH (2013) Intraoperative neurophysiologic monitoring and neurologic outcomes in patients with epidural spine tumors. Clin Neurol Neurosurg 115:2147–2152. doi:10.1016/j.clineuro.2013.08.008
2. Bozinov O, Burkhardt JK, Fischer CM, Kockro RA, Bernays RL, Bertalanffy H (2011) Advantages and limitations of intraoperative 3D ultrasound in neurosurgery. Technical note. Acta Neurochir Suppl 109:191–196. doi:10.1007/978-3-211-99651-5_30
3. Bozinov O, Burkhardt JK, Woernle CM, Hagel V, Ulrich NH, Krayenbühl N, Bertalanffy H (2012) Intra-operative high frequency ultrasound improves surgery of intramedullary cavernous malformations. Neurosurg Rev 35:269–275 (discussion 275)
4. Chadduck WM, Flanigan S (1985) Intraoperative ultrasound for spinal lesions. Neurosurgery 16:477–483
5. Cooper PR, Epstein F (1985) Radical resection of intramedullary spinal cord tumors in adults. Recent experience in 29 patients. J Neurosurg 63(4):492–499. doi:10.3171/jns.1985.63.4.0492
6. Costa P, Peretta P, Faccani G (2013) Relevance of intraoperative D wave in spine and spinal cord surgeries. Eur Spine J 22:840–848. doi:10.1007/s00586-012-2576-5
7. Degreif J, Wenda K (1998) Ultrasound-guided spinal fracture repositioning. Surg Endosc 12(2):164–169
8. Dohrmann GJ, Rubin JM (1988) Cervical spondylosis and syringomyelia: suboptimal results, incomplete treatment, and the role of intraoperative ultrasound. Clin Neurosurg 34:378–388
9. Duong LM, McCarthy BJ, McLendon RE, Dolecek TA, Kruchko C, Douglas LL, Ajani UA (2012) Descriptive epidemiology of malignant and non-malignant primary spinal cord, spinal meninges, and cauda equina tumors, United States, 2004–2007. Cancer 118:4220–4227. doi:10.1002/cncr.27390
10. Epstein FJ, Farmer JP, Schneider SJ (1991) Intraoperative ultrasonography: an important surgical adjunct for intramedullary tumors. J Neurosurg 74:729–733. doi:10.3171/jns.1991.74.5.0729
11. Friedman JA, Atkinson JL, Lane JI (2000) Migration of an intraspinal schwannoma documented by intraoperative ultrasound: case report. Surg Neurol 54:455–457
12. Friedman JA, Wetjen NM, Atkinson JL (2003) Utility of intraoperative ultrasound for tumors of the cauda equina. Spine (Phila Pa 1976) 28:288–290; discussion 291. doi:10.1097/01.BRS.0000042271.75392.E4
13. Glasier CM, Chadduck WM, Burrows PE (1986) Diagnosis of diastematomyelia with high-resolution spinal ultrasound. Childs Nerv Syst 2(5):255–257
14. Haberland N, Ebmeier K, Hliscs R, Grnewald JP, Silbermann J, Steenbeck J, Nowak H, Kalff R (2000) Neuronavigation in surgery of intracranial and spinal tumors. J Cancer Res Clin Oncol 126:529–541
15. Hammoud MA, Ligon BL, elSouki R, Shi WM, Schomer DF, Sawaya R (1996) Use of intraoperative ultrasound for localizing tumors and determining the extent of resection: a comparative study with magnetic resonance imaging. J Neurosurg 84:737–741. doi:10.3171/jns.1996.84.5.0737
16. Henegar MM, Vollmer DG, Silbergeld DL (1996) Intraoperative transligamentous ultrasound in the evaluation of thoracic intraspinal disease. Technique. Spine (Phila Pa 1976) 21:124–127
17. Jenkinson MD, Simpson C, Nicholas RS, Miles J, Findlay GF, Pigott TJ (2006) Outcome predictors and complications in the management of intradural spinal tumours. Eur Spine J 15:203–210. doi:10.1007/s00586-005-0902-x
18. Jokich PM, Rubin JM, Dohrmann GJ (1984) Intraoperative ultrasonic evaluation of spinal cord motion. J Neurosurg 60:707–711. doi:10.3171/jns.1984.60.4.0707
19. Kane RA, Kruskal JB (2007) Intraoperative ultrasonography of the brain and spine. Ultrasound Q 23:23–39. doi:10.1097/01.ruq.0000263840.92560.72
20. Koivukangas J, Tervonen O (1989) Intraoperative ultrasound imaging in lumbar disc herniation surgery. Acta Neurochir (Wien) 98:47–54
21. Koivukangas J, Tervonen O, Alasaarela E, Ylitalo J, Nyström S (1989) Completely computer-focused ultrasound imaging. First clinical imaging results. J Ultrasound Med 8:675–683
22. Kolstad F, Rygh OM, Selbekk T, Unsgaard G, Nygaard OP (2006) Three-dimensional ultrasonography navigation in spinal cord tumor surgery. Technical note. J Neurosurg Spine 5:264–270. doi:10.3171/spi.2006.5.3.264

23. Küllmer K, Eysel P, Rompe JD, Degreif J (1996) Intraoperative ultrasound in lumbar intervertebral disk displacement. Ultraschall Med 17(6):295–8
24. Lerch K, Völk M, Heers G, Baer W, Nerlich M (2002) Ultrasound-guided decompression of the spinal canal in traumatic stenosis. Ultrasound Med Biol 28(1):27–32
25. Maiuri F, Iaconetta G, de Divitiis O (1997) The role of intraoperative sonography in reducing invasiveness during surgery for spinal tumors. Minim Invasive Neurosurg 40:8–12. doi:10.1055/s-2008-1053405
26. Maiuri F, Iaconetta G, Gallicchio B, Stella L (2000) Intraoperative sonography for spinal tumors. Correlations with MR findings and surgery. J Neurosurg Sci 44:115–122
27. Nagelhus Hernes TA, Lindseth F, Selbekk T, Wollf A, Solberg OV, Harg E, Rygh OM, Tangen GA, Rasmussen I, Augdal S, Couweleers F, Unsgaard G (2006) Computer-assisted 3D ultrasound-guided neurosurgery: technological contributions, including multimodal registration and advanced display, demonstrating future perspectives. Int J Med Robot 2:45–59. doi:10.1002/rcs.68
28. Onik GM (2000) Percutaneous diskectomy in the treatment of herniated lumbar disks. Neuroimaging Clin N Am 10(3):597–607
29. Platt JF, Rubin JM, Chandler WF, Bowerman RA, DiPietro MA (1988) Intraoperative spinal sonography in the evaluation of intramedullary tumors. J Ultrasound Med 7:317–325
30. Prada F, Del Bene M, Mattei L, Casali C, Filippini A, Legnani F, Mangraviti A, Saladino A, Perin A, Richetta C, Vetrano I, Moiraghi A, Saini M, DiMeco F (2014) Fusion imaging for intra-operative ultrasound-based navigation in neurosurgery. J Ultrasound 17(3):243–251. doi:10.1007/s40477-014-0111-8
31. Prada F, Del Bene M, Mattei L, Lodigiani L, DeBeni S, Kolev V, Vetrano I, Solbiati L, Sakas G, DiMeco F (2014) Preoperative magnetic resonance and intraoperative ultrasound fusion imaging for real-time neuronavigation in brain tumor surgery. Ultraschall Med. doi:10.1055/s-0034-1385347
32. Prada F, Perin A, Martegani A, Aiani L, Solbiati L, Lamperti M, Casali C, Legnani F, Mattei L, Saladino A, Saini M, DiMeco F (2014c) Intraoperative contrast-enhanced ultrasound for brain tumor surgery. Neurosurgery 74(5):542–552; discussion 552. doi:10.1227/NEU.0000000000000301
33. Prada F, Vetrano IG, Filippini A, Del Bene M, Perin A, Casali C, Legnani F, Saini M, DiMeco F (2014) Intraoperative ultrasound in spinal tumor surgery. J Ultrasound 17:195–202. doi:10.1007/s40477-014-0102-9
34. Rasmussen IA, Lindseth F, Rygh OM, Berntsen EM, Selbekk T, Xu J, Nagelhus Hernes TA, Harg E, Håberg A, Unsgaard G (2007) Functional neuronavigation combined with intra-operative 3D ultrasound: initial experiences during surgical resections close to eloquent brain areas and future directions in automatic brain shift compensation of preoperative data. Acta Neurochir (Wien) 149:365–378. doi:10.1007/s00701-006-1110-0
35. Regelsberger J, Fritzsche E, Langer N, Westphal M (2005) Intraoperative sonography of intra- and extramedullary tumors. Ultrasound Med Biol 31:593–598. doi:10.1016/j.ultrasmedbio.2005.01.016
36. Reid MH (1978) Ultrasonic visualization of a cervical cord cystic astrocytoma. AJR Am J Roentgenol 131:907–908. doi:10.2214/ajr.131.5.907
37. Rhodes DW, Bishop PA (1997) A review of diagnostic ultrasound of the spine and soft tissue. J Manipulative Physiol Ther 20:267–273
38. Rubin JM, Chandler WF (1987) The use of ultrasound during spinal cord surgery. World J Surg 11:570–578
39. Sandalcioglu IE, Gasser T, Asgari S, Lazorisak A, Engelhorn T, Egelhof T, Stolke D, Wiedemayer H (2005) Functional outcome after surgical treatment of intramedullary spinal cord tumors: experience with 78 patients. Spinal Cord 43:34–41. doi:10.1038/sj.sc.3101668
40. Schellinger KA, Propp JM, Villano JL, McCarthy BJ (2008) Descriptive epidemiology of primary spinal cord tumors. J Neurooncol 87:173–179. doi:10.1007/s11060-007-9507-z
41. Selbekk T, Jakola AS, Solheim O, Johansen TF, Lindseth F, Reinertsen I, Unsgård G (2013) Ultrasound imaging in neurosurgery: approaches to minimize surgically induced image artefacts for improved resection control. Acta Neurochir (Wien) 155:973–980
42. Shamov T, Eftimov T, Kaprelyan A, Enchev Y (2013) Ultrasound-based neuronavigation and spinal cord tumour surgery – marriage of convenience or notified incompatibility? Turk Neurosurg 23:329–335. doi:10.5137/1019-5149.JTN.6639-12.2
43. Theodotou BC, Powers SK (1986) Use of intraoperative ultrasound in decision making during spinal operations. Neurosurgery 19:205–211
44. Traul DE, Shaffrey ME, Schiff D (2007) Part I: spinal-cord neoplasms-intradural neoplasms. Lancet Oncol 8:35–45. doi:10.1016/S1470-2045(06)71009-9
45. Uff CE, Garcia L, Fromageau J, Dorward N, Bamber JC (2009) Real-time ultrasound elastography in neurosurgery. In, vol Proceedings of the IEEE International Ultrasonics Symposium. Proceedings of the IEEE International Ultrasonics Symposium. pp 467–470. doi:10.1109/ULTSYM.2009.0115
46. Zhou H, Miller D, Schulte DM, Benes L, Bozinov O, Sure U, Bertalanffy H (2011) Intraoperative ultrasound assistance in treatment of intradural spinal tumours. Clin Neurol Neurosurg 113:531–537. doi:10.1016/j.clineuro.2011.03.006

Intraoperative Findings in Peripheral Nerve Pathologies

Ralph W. Koenig, Jan Coburger, and Maria Teresa Pedro

7.1 Introduction

For many years, intraoperative B-mode ultrasound has been part of the clinical routine in cranial and spinal neurosurgery, mainly for localization and resection control [3, 4, 21, 24]. In peripheral nerve surgery, intraoperative application of ultrasound did not play any role so far, primarily because of the technical demands warranted to visualize peripheral nerves and peripheral nerve pathologies. Nowadays, as a consequence of an ongoing software and transducer development, high-frequency, high-resolution ultrasound of peripheral nerves from its first description by Fornage [9] became a highly versatile tool in the diagnostic work-up of peripheral nerve pathologies: entrapment, trauma, tumor, and neuropathies [13, 22].

The first intraoperative application of high-resolution ultrasound in peripheral nerve surgery was described by Lee et al. [17]. Usage was mainly limited to correct localization of different nerves and nerve pathologies and based on this, planning of the surgical approach and skin inci-

R.W. Koenig (✉) • J. Coburger • M.T. Pedro
Department of Neurosurgery, University of Ulm,
Ludwig-Heilmeyerstr. 3, 89312 Günzburg, Germany
e-mail: ralph.koenig@uni-ulm.de;
jan.coburger@uni-ulm.de;
maria-teresa.pedro@uni-ulm.de

sion. Thereafter, our study group [14] described a technique for direct intraoperative high-resolution ultrasound of exposed peripheral nerves, taking advantage of its tissue differentiating properties to assess the type and degree of neural fibrosis in traumatic nerve lesions.

7.2 Clinical Application

7.2.1 Localization and Planning of Surgical Approach

Exposure of peripheral nerves especially in trauma and tumor surgery so far was characterized by extensive surgical exposures. The main reason for this was a lack of morphological information about the affected nerve, especially in traumatic nerve surgery. Even with continuous improvements in peripheral nerve imaging, mainly MRI and high-resolution ultrasound [1, 6, 13, 20, 23], transposing the imaging information into the operative situs turns out to be difficult frequently. Therefore, implementation of high-quality imaging in peripheral nerve surgery together with endoscopic techniques [11, 16] allowed targeted approaches and exposures of peripheral nerves. These developments in nerve surgery led to tailored surgical exposures with the advantage of less tissue trauma.

© Springer International Publishing Switzerland 2016
F. Prada et al. (eds.), *Intraoperative Ultrasound (IOUS) in Neurosurgery:*
From Standard B-mode to Elastosonography, DOI 10.1007/978-3-319-25268-1_7

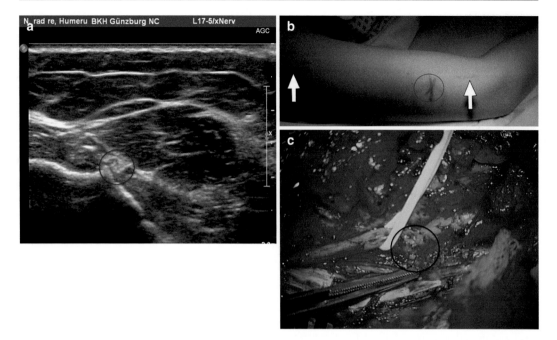

Fig. 7.1 (**a–c**) (**a**) Preoperative cross-sectional ultrasound (17–5 MHz linear array probe) depicting the radial nerve adjacent to a bony spur. (**b**) Intraoperative photo of the affected upper arm before sterile draping. The area of interest (*red circle*) was localized using intraoperative ultrasound; *white arrows* pointing out the preexisting scars after humerus nailing. (**c**) Intraoperative microscope image after tailored approach centered over the suspicious nerve segment: radial nerve markedly scarred to the humeral bone spur (*black circle*)

Case 7.1 (See Fig. 7.1a–c)

A 22-year-old female patient presented with typical radial nerve palsy after humerus fracture with consecutive nailing 3 months ago. She presented with a complete drop hand and missing clinical and electrophysiological signs of spontaneous recovery. On preoperative ultrasound, a major nerve lesion could be excluded; there was suspicion of circumscribed radial nerve compression at the distal end of the spiral groove, due to an exophytic bone spur. With the aid of intraoperative ultrasound, the affected nerve segment could be exposed via a tailored surgical approach centered over the conspicuous area. The nerve was found to be adherent at the bone spur and markedly scarred. After external microsurgical neurolysis, intraoperative CNAPs (compound nerve action potentials) could be recorded over the affected nerve segment. Thus, further spontaneous regeneration could be expected, and nerve grafting was not required.

7.2.2 Tissue Differentiation in Trauma and Tumor Surgery

The unsurpassed spatial resolution of high-frequency linear-array ultrasound allows for depiction of least tissue details in peripheral nerves, e.g., its internal structure, epineurium, and fascicles [12–14, 18]. Due to its restricted tissue penetration, this tissue differentiating property of high-frequency ultrasound can only be utilized in superficially located nerves. In order to overcome these technical restrictions, direct examination of surgically exposed peripheral nerves was developed [14]. For this, the nerve segment involved is externally neurolysed and embedded in sterile ultrasound gel cushions, which serve as an offset spacer. In near-field ultrasound (e.g., in dermatology), offset spacers are routinely used to bring the objects into the optimal distance to the probe aperture. Thereby, image quality is improved.

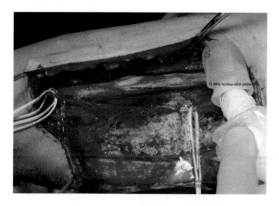

Fig. 7.2 Intraoperative photo illustrating the technique of intraoperative ultrasound of peripheral nerves. Scanning of the median nerve at right upper arm level. The nerve is embedded in a gel cushion. The high-frequency linear array ultrasound (15–7 MHz, linear array, hockey stick, small footprint) probe is directly applied on the nerve

Furthermore, those gel cushions serve as an excellent couplant, and deformation artifacts induced with direct application of the transducer on the nerve are reduced (Fig. 7.2).

7.2.2.1 Trauma

Neuromas-in-continuity account for the most frequent traumatic peripheral nerve lesions [10]. Their management is often challenging, especially in cases with partial functional recovery. Often the extent of nerve damage cannot be assessed preoperatively. Even with surgical exposure and palpation of the affected nerve segment, correct assessment of the underlying injury remains difficult, as nerve lesions of similar external appearance might harbor completely different pathological features: complete lesions which have to be resected and grafted or lesions that contain enough prevailing conducting fascicular structures to enable spontaneous functional regeneration. Intraoperative high-resolution ultrasound enables nerve surgeons to have a look inside the damaged nerve segment [14] and to judge their injury based on changes in the outer diameter, assessment of internal architecture, and extent of fibrosis. A simple classification system derived therefrom shows very high correlation with intraoperative nerve-action-potential recordings and

histopathology and therefore serves as decisive support for the intraoperative management of neuromas-in-continuity (Table 7.1).

Case 7.2

A 70-year-old lady fractured her right elbow and suffered an incomplete median nerve lesion. She presented 5 months after trauma. Despite intensive physiotherapy, spontaneous recovery was unsatisfying, although she was able to flex her index finger (flexor digitorum superficialis Dig II., M4). After surgical exposure, the median nerve was found partially lesioned. An ultrasound-guided intraneural dissection led to resection and grafting of partial neuroma-in-continuity. Intact nerve fascicles correlating to the preserved function after trauma were spared (Figs. 7.3 and 7.4).

7.2.2.2 Tumors

There is a certain dilemma associated with the preoperative diagnosis of peripheral nerve tumors and tumor-like lesions. Even differential diagnosis between the most common peripheral nerve tumors [15], schwannomas and neurofibromas, is not as trivial as it first appears. Especially differentiation from malignant peripheral nerve sheath tumors (MPNST) despite advanced imaging modalities like MR neurography and PET is not possible yet [2, 5, 7, 8]. But since their clinical and surgical management differs widely, direct intraoperative high-resolution ultrasound with its tissue differentiating properties may support the intraoperative surgical decision-making process. So far, only preliminary experience concerning intraoperative high-resolution and contrast-enhanced ultrasound (CEUS) in peripheral nerve tumor surgery is available. But according to our limited experience so far, ultrasound, especially CEUS, might be an additional piece in the mosaic to help at least intraoperative differentiation between benign and malignant tumors [19]. Therefore, besides intraoperative localization and approach planning, ultrasound might be able to give decisive information about the nature of the underlying pathology of nerve tumors or tumor-like lesions.

Table 7.1 Classification of nerve injuries based on intraoperative high-resolution ultrasound

	Normal	Epineural fibrosis	Intraneural fibrosis	Partial neuroma-in-continuity	Complete neuroma-in-continuity
	I	II	III	IV	V
Outer diameter	Normal	Normal, partly mild swelling	Normal, partly mild swelling	Fusiform swelling	Fusiform swelling
Internal architecture	Honeycomb pattern	Honeycomb pattern	Preserved hypoechogenic fascicular structures, increase of hyperechogenic tissue, reduced differentiation	Cross section containing compartments of preserved honeycomb pattern beneath hyperechogenic neuroma	Missing, hyperechogenic tissue
Fibrosis	Missing	Epineural	Epineural merging to intraneural fibrosis	Different compartments	Fibrosis of complete cross section
CNAP recordings	Normal	Normal, especially after epineurotomy	Reduced amplitude of CNAP	Depending on the compartment	CNAP negative
Prognosis/therapy	Good prognosis	Epineurotomy Good prognosis	Intraneural dissection with partial epineural resection	Split repair	Grafting

CNAP compound nerve action potential

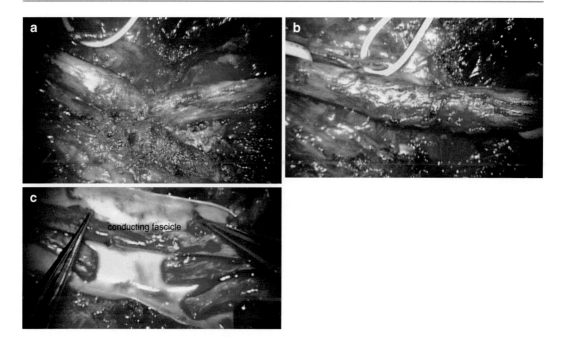

Fig. 7.3 (**a–c**) Intraoperative microscopic images illustrating the surgical steps in case 2: (**a**) median nerve retracted into the humeral fracture gap. (**b**) After external neurolysis, the nerve is in continuity. (**c**) After interfascicular dissection, resection of partial neuroma in continuity and preparation for split repair

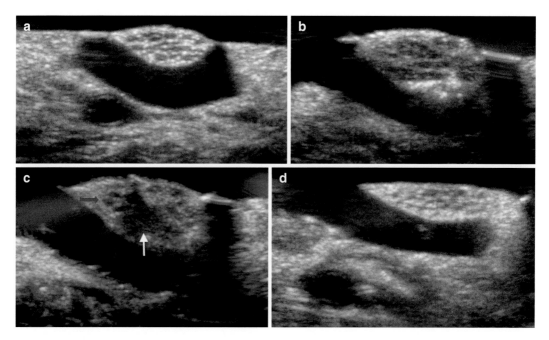

Fig. 7.4 (**a–d**) Intraoperative ultrasound (15–7 MHz linear array probe) case 2: (**a**) median nerve after external neurolysis, embedded in sterile hydrogel. Proximal to the lesion: depiction of typical honeycomb-like fascicular nerve structure. (**b**) Proximal nerve segment adjacent to the lesion: enlarged cross section, signs of epineural fibrosis and irregular intrinsic echotexture. (**c**) Over the lesion: partial neuroma (*white arrow*) beneath some intact fascicular structures (*red arrow*). (**d**) Intact nerve structure distal to the lesion

Example 1

Schwannoma of the tibial nerve at the popliteal
fossa (Fig. 7.5a–b)

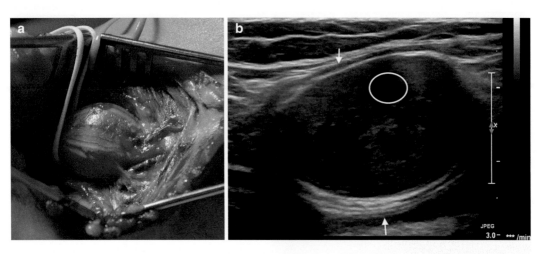

Fig. 7.5 (**a–b**) (**a**) Intraoperative photo: surgical site of tibial nerve schwannoma exposed at the level of the popliteal fossa. (**b**) Corresponding longitudinal section of intraoperative ultrasound (17–5 MHz linear array probe) depicting the typical appearance of a schwannoma: an isoechogenic to hypoechogenic tumor, often with cystic components (*white circle*). The nerve fascicles passing marginal to the tumor (*white arrows*)

Example 2
Amyloidoma of the peroneal nerve (Fig. 7.6a–e)

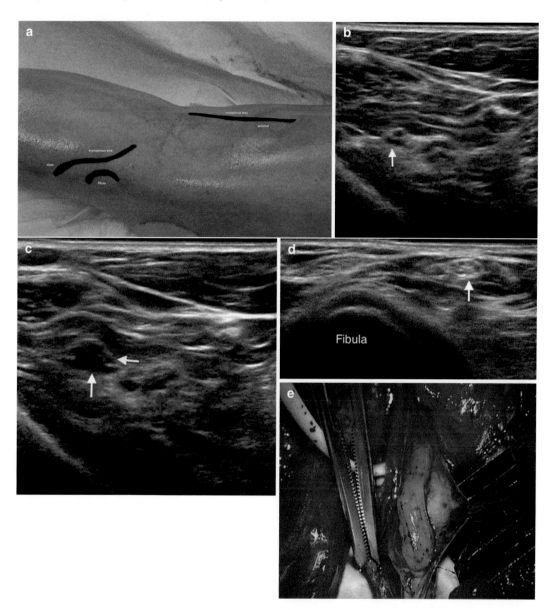

Fig. 7.6 (a–e) (a) Intraoperative photo of right leg at the level of the poplitea. Planned skin incision for peroneal nerve exposure. (b) Intraoperative ultrasound (17–5 MHz, linear array probe) at distal thigh depicting the peroneal (*white arrow*) and tibial (*red arrow*) nerve with normal echotexture. (c). Intraoperative ultrasound at popliteal level. Cross section of the peroneal nerve appears markedly enlarged; one hypoechogenic, swollen fascicle is noticeable (*white arrow*), while the remaining nerve appears normal (*yellow arrow*). Medially, the tibial nerve is depicted (*red arrow*). (d) Intraoperative ultrasound at the level of the fibula with intact fascicular structure of perineal nerve (*white arrow*). (e) Intraoperative photo demonstrating the corresponding enlarged fascicle after interfascicular dissection. Histopathological examination revealed an amyloidoma

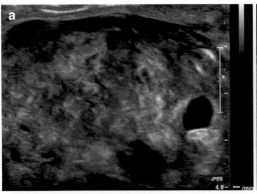 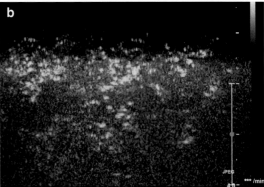

Fig. 7.7 (**a**, **b**) (**a**) Intraoperative ultrasound (12–5 MHz linear array probe, capable of CEUS) depicting a solid, partially cystic tumor mass, with an uneasy tissue structure; normal nerve structure marginal to or inside the

lesion cannot be depicted. (**b**) Intraoperative CEUS after application of 4.8 ml SonoVue® reveals strong tumor perfusion. A positive perfusion pattern was depicted after 21 s increasing diffusely over the next 38 s

Example 3
Example of MPNST of the sciatic nerve (Fig. 7.7a, b)

References

1. Breckwoldt MO, Stock C, Xia A, Heckel A, Bendszus M, Pham M, Heiland S, Bäumer P (2015) Diffusion tensor imaging adds diagnostic accuracy in magnetic resonance neurography. Invest Radiol 1:498–504. doi:10.1097/RLI.0000000000000156
2. Capek S, Hébert-Blouin M-N, Puffer RC, Martinoli C, Frick MA, Amrami KK, Spinner RJ (2015) Tumefactive appearance of peripheral nerve involvement in hematologic malignancies: a new imaging association. Skeletal Radiol 44:1001–1009. doi:10.1007/s00256-015-2151-3
3. Coburger J, König RW, Scheuerle A, Engelke J, Hlavac M, Thal DR, Wirtz CR (2014) Navigated high frequency ultrasound: description of technique and clinical comparison with conventional intracranial ultrasound. World Neurosurg 82:366–375. doi:10.1016/j.wneu.2014.05.025
4. Coburger J, Scheuerle A, Thal DR, Engelke J, Hlavac M, Wirtz CR, König R (2015) Linear array ultrasound in low-grade glioma surgery: histology-based assessment of accuracy in comparison to conventional intraoperative ultrasound and intraoperative MRI. Acta Neurochir 157:195–206. doi:10.1007/s00701-014-2314-3
5. Consales A, Roncaroli F, Salvi F, Poppi M (2003) Amyloidoma of the brachial plexus. Surg Neurol 59:418–423; discussion 423
6. Coraci D, Tsukamoto H, Granata G, Briani C, Santilli V, Padua L (2015) Fibular nerve damage in knee dislocation: spectrum of ultrasound patterns. Muscle Nerve 51:859–863. doi:10.1002/mus.24472
7. Descamps MJL, Barrett L, Groves M, Yung L, Birch R, Murray NMF, Linch DC, Lunn MPT, Reilly MM (2006) Primary sciatic nerve lymphoma: a case report and review of the literature. J Neurol Neurosurg Psychiatry 77:1087–1089. doi:10.1136/jnnp.2006.087577
8. Ferner RE, Golding JF, Smith M, Calonje E, Jan W, Sanjayanathan V, O'Doherty M (2008) [18 F]2-fluoro-2-deoxy-D-glucose positron emission tomography (FDG PET) as a diagnostic tool for neurofibromatosis 1 (NF1) associated malignant peripheral nerve sheath tumours (MPNSTs): a long-term clinical study. Ann Oncol 19:390–394. doi:10.1093/annonc/mdm450
9. Fornage BD (1988) Peripheral nerves of the extremities: imaging with US. Radiology 167:179–182. doi:10.1148/radiology.167.1.3279453
10. Friedman AH (2009) An eclectic review of the history of peripheral nerve surgery. Neurosurgery 65:A3–A8. doi:10.1227/01.NEU.0000346252.53722.D3
11. Giuliano Heinen CP, Schmidt T, Kretschmer T (2015) Endoscopically assisted piriformis-to-knee surgery of sciatic, peroneal, and tibial nerves: technical note. Neurosurgery 11(Suppl 2):37–42; discussion 42. doi:10.1227/NEU.0000000000000621
12. Kermarrec E, Demondion X, Khalil C, Le Thuc V, Boutry N, Cotten A (2010) Ultrasound and magnetic resonance imaging of the peripheral nerves: current techniques, promising directions, and open issues.

Semin Musculoskelet Radiol 14:463–472. doi:10.105 5/s-0030-1268067

13. Koenig RW, Pedro MT, Heinen CPG, Schmidt T, Richter H-P, Antoniadis G, Kretschmer T (2009) High-resolution ultrasonography in evaluating peripheral nerve entrapment and trauma. Neurosurg Focus 26:E13. doi:10.3171/FOC.2009.26.2.E13

14. Koenig RW, Schmidt TE, Heinen CPG, Wirtz CR, Kretschmer T, Antoniadis G, Pedro MT (2011) Intraoperative high-resolution ultrasound: a new technique in the management of peripheral nerve disorders. J Neurosurg 114:514–521. doi:10.3171/2010.9. JNS10464

15. Kransdorf MJ (1995) Benign soft-tissue tumors in a large referral population: distribution of specific diagnoses by age, sex, and location. AJR Am J Roentgenol 164:395–402. doi:10.2214/ajr.164.2.7839977

16. Krishnan KG, Pinzer T, Reber F, Schackert G (2004) Endoscopic exploration of the brachial plexus: technique and topographic anatomy--a study in fresh human cadavers. Neurosurgery 54:401–408; discussion 408–409

17. Lee FC, Singh H, Nazarian LN, Ratliff JK (2011) High-resolution ultrasonography in the diagnosis and intraoperative management of peripheral nerve lesions. J Neurosurg 114:206–211. doi:10.3171/2010. 2.JNS091324

18. Padua L, Granata G, Sabatelli M, Inghilleri M, Lucchetta M, Luigetti M, Coraci D, Martinoli C, Briani C (2014) Heterogeneity of root and nerve ultrasound pattern in CIDP patients. Clin Neurophysiol 125:160–165. doi:10.1016/j.clinph.2013.07.023

19. Pedro MT, Antoniadis G, Scheuerle A, Pham M, Wirtz CR, Koenig RW (2015) Intraoperative high-resolution ultrasound (IHRU) and contrast enhanced ultrasound (ICEUS) in peripheral nerve tumors and tumor-like lesions. Neurosurg Focus 39(3):E5. doi:1 0.3171/2015.6.FOCUS15218

20. Pham M, Bäumer T, Bendszus M (2014) Peripheral nerves and plexus: imaging by MR-neurography and high-resolution ultrasound. Curr Opin Neurol 27:370–379. doi:10.1097/WCO.0000000000000111

21. Prada F, Vetrano IG, Filippini A, Del Bene M, Perin A, Casali C, Legnani F, Saini M, DiMeco F (2014) Intraoperative ultrasound in spinal tumor surgery. J Ultrasound 17:195–202. doi:10.1007/ s40477-014-0102-9

22. Shy ME (2015) Ultrasound: the future for evaluating the PNS in humans? J Neurol Neurosurg Psychiatry 86:362. doi:10.1136/jnnp-2014-308855

23. Simon NG, Spinner RJ, Kline DG, Kliot M (2015) Advances in the neurological and neurosurgical management of peripheral nerve trauma. J Neurol Neurosurg Psychiatr. jnnp–2014–310175. doi:10.1136/jnnp-2014-310175

24. Sosna J, Barth MM, Kruskal JB, Kane RA (2005) Intraoperative sonography for neurosurgery. J Ultrasound Med 24:1671–1682

Multimodal Imaging in Glioma Surgery

8

Andrej Šteňo, Carlo Giussani, and Matteo Riva

8.1 Neuronavigation and Intraoperative Magnetic Resonance Imaging in Glioma Surgery

Maximal safe resection positively influences prognosis of patients harboring infiltrative brain gliomas; the extent of tumor resection was proven to be a significant predictor of survival both in grade II gliomas (low-grade gliomas) and in grade III and IV gliomas (high-grade gliomas) [1, 2]. However, resections of these tumors are faced with the problem of macroscopic similarity of gliomas and the normal brain [3]. This problem is prominent mostly in grade II gliomas, which can be macroscopically "invisible" [3], despite the magnification of surgical microscope.

Because gliomas are usually well visualized by magnetic resonance imaging (MRI), neuronavigation utilizing preoperative 3D MRI sequences is used in many centers in order to localize the tumor tissue (Fig. 8.1) [4–10]. Several

different neuronavigation systems based on similar principle have been developed in the last decades. Briefly, after the head of the patient is fixed on the surgical table, the position of the head is co-registered together with the preoperative MRI image set; subsequently, the tip of a specific pointer (which is recognized by the neuronavigation system) is virtually reproduced on the preoperative MRI images. A significant impact of neuronavigation to achieve gross total resection of malignant brain gliomas was shown by retrospective analyses presented by Kurimoto et al. [5] and Wirtz et al. [4]. However, the prospective randomized study performed by Willems et al. failed to show any benefit of neuronavigation during resections of solitary intracerebral contrast-enhancing tumors as compared to standard surgery without neuronavigation [11]. One plausible explanation for the negative result might be the limited accuracy of neuronavigation, which is sufficient only before the brain-shift occurs, i.e., before the tumor resection. During the surgical procedure, the loss of cerebrospinal fluid, the progressive tumor removal, the use of retractors, and the brain edema constantly produce a shift of the position of brain structures, making the neuronavigation system so imprecise that it is no longer reliable [12]. Intraoperative imaging techniques – intraoperative MRI (iMRI) and navigated 3D-ultrasound – represent the solution to this problem, as they allow an update of the neuronavigation data during the surgical procedure.

A. Šteňo, MD, PhD (✉)
Department of Neurosurgery, Comenius University Faculty of Medicine, University Hospital Bratislava, Limbova 5, Bratislava, Slovakia
e-mail: andrej.steno@gmail.com

C. Giussani • M. Riva
Department of Neurosurgery,
University of Milano-Bicocca, San Gerardo University Hospital, Monza, Italy

© Springer International Publishing Switzerland 2016
F. Prada et al. (eds.), *Intraoperative Ultrasound (IOUS) in Neurosurgery:
From Standard B-mode to Elastosonography*, DOI 10.1007/978-3-319-25268-1_8

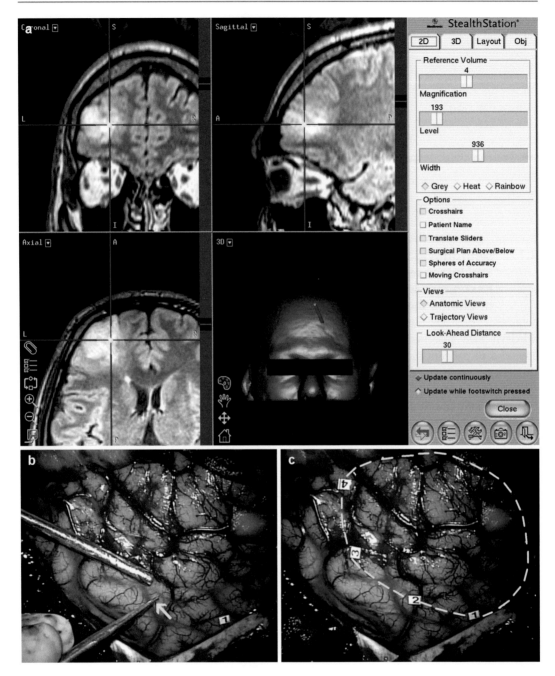

Fig. 8.1 (a) Oligodendroglioma grade II well depicted by preoperative 3D FLAIR MRI sequence, which was used for neuronavigation. (b, c) Neuronavigation had to be used to identify the tumor tissue, as it was not distinguishable from the surrounding brain (despite infiltration of the cortex). *Arrow*: tip of the pointer. *Numbers*: posterior (pseudo)border of the tumor. *Interrupted yellow line*: whole cortical part of the tumor (identified by neuronavigation). Surgery performed at the Department of Neurosurgery in Bratislava

Over the last 15 years, intraoperative magnetic resonance imaging (iMRI) gained increased attention as the first choice in intraoperative imaging. Starting from 0.5 T magnets, the iMRI evolved in two directions: (ultra)low-field iMRI and high-field iMRI. Ultralow-field usually refers to systems of 0.2 T or less, low-field to systems of around 0.5 T, and high-field to systems of at least 1.5 T.

Since the introduction of iMRI, different reports have been published supporting the utility of iMRI-guided surgery and its positive impact on extent of glioma resection (high-grade as well as low-grade gliomas) and patients survival using both low-field and high-field systems [13–21]. Despite the fact highlighted in two systematic reviews [22, 23] that only few studies are prospective and only one study is a randomized control trial, the evidence that iMRI has a positive influence in the treatment of patients with glioma is rather solid. In the solitary randomized controlled trial examining the impact of iMRI on extent of resection of glioblastoma patients published by Senft et al. [21], 58 patients were randomized to receive a standard versus iMRI-guided tumor removal, with an independent masked neuroradiologist doing the evaluation of preoperative and postoperative images. 49 patients were analyzed and 9 patients were excluded because of non-glial (metastatic) tumor at histology or they refused to randomization. In the iMRI group, the intraoperative scanning showed a tumor remnant leading to a further tumor removal in 33 % of cases, and the total resection was achieved in 96 % of patients, which was significantly higher comparing to 68 % of the control group. On multivariate analysis, the extent of resection was the only factor that affected progression-free survival [21].

In addition to the data confirming positive impact of iMRI on extent of glioma resection, the ability of intraoperative imaging to compensate the brain-shift can undisputedly increase the safety of surgery – considering the fact that important structures such as eloquent tracts can shift up to 15 mm [24].

However, besides clear benefits of iMRI, several drawbacks should also be mentioned. First, image quality of low- and ultralow-field systems is inferior comparing to high-field iMRI [25] and that predominantly in low-grade gliomas [25] but also in some benign lesions, e.g., pituitary adenomas [26]. Second, besides superior image quality, the implementation and maintenance costs of

high-field iMRI systems are much higher than in ultralow-field and low-field iMRI [25]; in addition, the costs of (ultra)low-field iMRI systems are significantly higher than in some other intraoperative imaging modalities such as intraoperative ultrasound [27]. Depending on the type of intraoperative MRI system, installation costs US$ 3–8 million [21]. Third, though high-field iMRI systems (unlike low-field systems) allow to perform advanced imaging techniques as diffusion tensor imaging and intraoperative tractography [28], the intraoperative reconstruction of white matter tracts is not always realizable [29]; electrophysiological neuromonitoring of eloquent subcortical structures is still the gold standard not replaceable by iMRI [29]. Last and most importantly, the prolongation of surgical procedure is significant when iMRI systems are used [30]. Despite that the acquisition times of high-field iMRI are shorter compared to low-field systems, for a proper evaluation, it is necessary to take into account not only the time necessary for performing the scans but also the prolonged time for patients' preparation before the surgical incision. If the whole occupation time of the operating room is considered, the difference between iMRI-guided and standard surgery increases about 60 min [21]. Obviously, if more than one iMRI scan is needed, the procedure is further significantly prolonged.

In view of these points, other alternative methods for intraoperative imaging and faster update of neuronavigation data may be considered, especially for guidance of procedures with limited surgical time, such as awake resections (AR) of brain gliomas.

8.2 Intraoperative Ultrasound in Glioma Surgery

8.2.1 Intraoperative 2D-Ultrasound in Glioma Surgery

In the early 1980s, the intraoperative use of B-mode 2D-ultrasound was introduced in order to visualize glioma tissue during neurosurgical procedures [31]. After more than 30 years of use,

2D-ultrasound was proven to be a valuable, truly real-time intraoperative imaging tool that can guide neurosurgeons in decision making and surgical planning [32].

Despite significant benefits of 2D-ultrasound during glioma surgery however, several pitfalls were recognized that prevented 2D-ultrasound from becoming a major breakthrough [33].

Image quality The main disadvantage of older 2D-ultrasound systems was low image quality [34], due to poor spatial resolution and dynamic range. Differentiation of various brain structures was challenging and required extensive experience. Nevertheless, the imaging quality is certainly influenced by the ultrasound system used, and many new ultrasound systems have much improved quality. One of the improvements to image quality is due to the ability of modern ultrasound systems to electronically and dynamically tune the frequency range of the imaging

probe [35]. Higher frequency means better resolution, i.e., a better ability to differentiate two targets as separate objects [35]. High-frequency linear array ultrasound showed a significant benefit for residual glioblastoma detection in comparison with the lower-frequency curved array ultrasound [36]. For low-grade gliomas, the accuracy of residual tumor detection is comparable to high-field intraoperative MRI when a high-frequency ultrasound linear probe is used [37]. However, the drawback of high-frequency probes is the reduced penetration of acoustic waves in the tissue [35]. As recommended by Unsgaard et al. [38], to obtain the best image, different probes should be used for imaging of lesions localized in different depths (Fig. 8.2). A 5 MHz (4–8 MHz) probe gives optimal image quality at a distance of 2.5–6 cm from the probe, while for superficial lesions ,a 12 MHz linear probe is ideal as it produces the best image quality for the first few millimeters down to a depth of 4 cm [38].

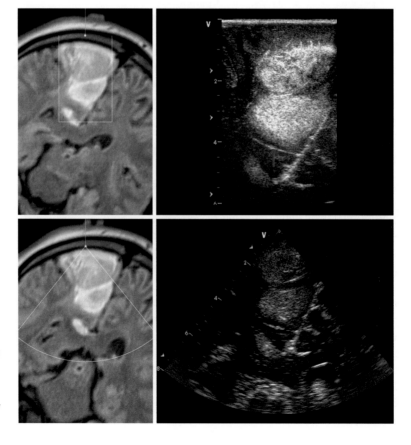

Fig. 8.2 Bicentric grade II astrocytoma. *Upper row*: Visualization of the superficial tumor with 12 MHz linear probe. Note that the sulcus under the tumor (*red arrow*) is not visible on 1.5 T 3D-FLAIR sequence. *Lower row*: Visualization of the deeper tumor with 8 MHz phased array probe. Note distinct visualization of the (pseudo) border between the deeper tumor and corpus callosum. Surgery performed at the Department of Neurosurgery in Bratislava

As evaluated by histopathology, a high-end intraoperative ultrasound system was proven to depict glioma (pseudo)borders at least as good as a T2-weighted MRI image and better than a T1-weighted MRI image [39]. Both low-grade and high-grade glioma tissue are well visualized by ultrasound [39–42]; however, in patients who had received radiotherapy, the quality of imaging may decrease [42].

Artifacts A well-known drawback of every ultrasound device is ultrasound artifacts [43–45]. The most prominent problem is the acoustic enhancement artifacts (AEAs) that appear at the bottom of the resection cavity after some tumor debulking [40, 46], when ultrasound penetrates through a higher column of water (saline). The appearance of AEAs is due to a large difference between a very low attenuation of acoustic waves in saline and high attenuation of acoustic waves in brain tissue [46, 47]. The ultrasonic depiction of medial tumor borders after some tumor debulking may therefore be problematic [44]; AEAs may even preclude the detection of tumor remnants at the bottom of the resection cavity. However, there are several methods available to differentiate between AEAs and tumor remnants and estimate the extent of resection.

The first possibility is simply to move the probe. In real-time 2D-ultrasound, the location of the AEAs in the image will move when the probe is moved or altered in position and angle [46].

Another possibility to indirectly distinguish AEAs and residual tumor is comparison between pre-resectional and updated ultrasound image, performed during or after resection. If the hyperechoic area is localized in a region where no tumor was present before the resection, it is most probably not a tumor remnant [48].

AEAs may be minimized also by inserting a miniature ultrasound probe into the resection cavity [36, 40, 46, 48, 49]. By doing so, the column of water between the tip of the miniature probe and scanned tissue at the bottom of resection cavity is smaller than when scanning with a larger probe placed on the brain surface. Shortening the column of water reduces the AEAs at the bottom of resection cavity; the struc-

tures in the medial part of resection cavity can be distinctly depicted (Fig. 8.3).

A new potential possibility of minimizing the AEAs is by utilizing the artifact-reducing acoustic coupling fluid. This fluid was developed recently by the group of G. Unsgaard [46, 47].

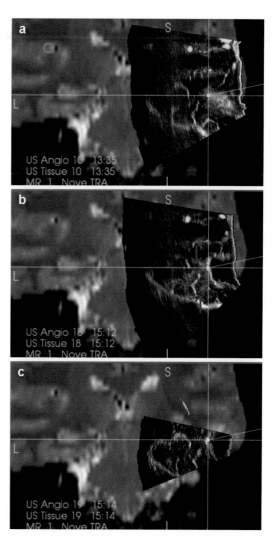

Fig. 8.3 Small temporal grade II oligodendroglioma. (**a**) Initial ultrasound image scanned from the dural surface fused with the preoperative navigation MRI. (**b**) Ultrasound scan performed from the dural surface after the tumor resection. Note distinct depiction of brain structures alongside the resection cavity and the bright artifact at the bottom of the resection cavity (*arrows*). (**c**) Ultrasound image acquired with mini-probe inserted within the resection cavity. Note minimization of the artifact; no tumor remnant is present. Surgery performed at the Department of Neurosurgery in Bratislava

Because the coupling fluid attenuates ultrasound energy like normal brain tissue, the AEAs are minimized. A phase 1 clinical study where different concentrations of the acoustic coupling fluid are being tested in selected patients is ongoing [47].

Oblique views Most neurosurgeons have extensive experience with the interpretation of MRI images in three orthogonal planes – axial, coronal, and sagittal. However, they usually have little or no experience with the interpretation of intraoperative 2D-ultrasound views that are mostly oblique [50]. In addition, an ultrasound probe has a limited field of view; it is possible to evaluate only a section of brain tissue during real-time 2D-ultrasound scanning. Due to this reason, the orientation problem has always been considerable for many surgeons [51]. The interpretation of 2D-ultrasound image is difficult particularly in areas with no cysts or ventricles visible [50]. Consequently, after introduction of frameless neuronavigation that shows brain and pathological tissue in "classic" three orthogonal planes, many neurosurgeons preferred the use of navigation for glioma surgery guidance [4–10]. In addition, unlike 2D-ultrasound, neuronavigation is effective also in planning the craniotomy placement. On the other hand, because navigation can become significantly inaccurate after the occurrence of brain-shift [28], the intraoperative utilization of 2D-ultrasound, which is a real-time imaging device, continued in numerous centers [52–57].

8.2.2 Navigated 3D-ultrasound in Glioma Surgery

In order to merge the advantages and overcome the disadvantages of both stand-alone 2D-ultrasound and neuronavigation devices, some groups have connected ultrasound scanner to conventional neuronavigation, digitized the analog video signal from the scanner, and displayed a real-time 2D-ultrasound image on the navigation computer side by side with the corresponding MRI slice [58–60]. This solution simplified the interpretation of ultrasound imagery and allowed quantification of brain-shift [61].

Nevertheless, a major step forward presented later was the integration of neuronavigation and ultrasound devices based on a digital interface between the ultrasound scanner and the navigation computer. Such integration was the basis for the development of navigated 3D-ultrasound – a system that enables neuronavigation using 3D-ultrasound data as well as preoperative MRI [61]. Modern navigated 3D-ultrasound devices dedicated to neurosurgery allow intraoperative ultrasound image rendering in three orthogonal planes and automatic fusion with navigation MRI sequence. By combining frameless navigation with 3D-ultrasound, these systems solve the most prominent drawbacks of 2D-ultrasound and conventional neuronavigation – namely, the orientation and brain-shift problems [51]. Rendering the ultrasound image in axial, coronal, and sagittal planes makes the recognition of normal and glioma infiltrated brain structures much more easy [62] (Fig. 8.4). In addition, navigated 3D-ultrasound provides almost real-time imaging and allows re-scanning of the operating field as often as necessary [51].

3D-ultrasound devices allow for a more straightforward way of dealing with the artifacts. These systems allow comparison of pre-resectional and updated images in all three planes; based on this comparison, it is possible to indirectly evaluate the presence or absence of glioma remnants (Fig. 8.5). In the case where a 3D-ultrasound device equipped with a miniature probe is used, the 3D-ultrasound data can be acquired with the mini-probe inserted into the resection cavity (Figs. 8.5 and 8.6). This method was presented by Steno et al. [40] and its efficacy was confirmed by the group of G. Unsgaard [46].

Another advantage of navigated 3D-ultrasound and 2D-ultrasound is the cost, which is significantly lower than the price of intraoperative MRI. In addition, implementation of ultrasound into the operating room is easier, since no special infrastructural or instrumental adaptations are needed.

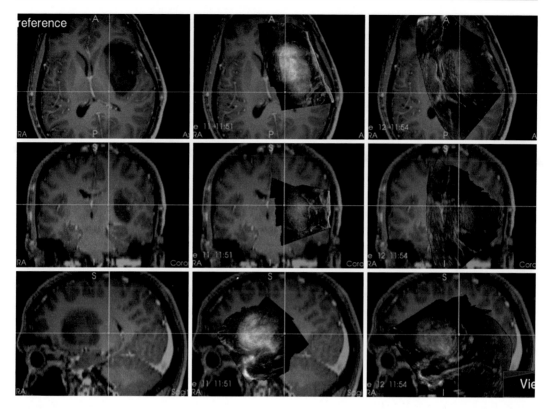

Fig. 8.4 Right-sided insular astrocytoma. *Left column*: Preoperative contrast-enhanced 3D T1 MRI navigation sequence. *Middle column*: 3D-ultrasound image acquired with 12 MHz linear probe fused with navigation MRI. Note better visualization of superficial structures. *Right column*: 3D-ultrasound image acquired with 8 MHz phased array probe fused with navigation MRI. Note better visualization of deep structures. Surgery performed at the Department of Neurosurgery in Bratislava

8.2.3 Intraoperative Ultrasound during Awake Resection of Brain Gliomas

Diffuse gliomas may infiltrate and incorporate functionally important brain structures [63, 64], which makes the resection of tumors localized to eloquent areas challenging. Despite the progress in visualization of eloquent cortex and white matter tracts by functional MRI and tractography based on diffusion tensor imaging, these modalities are not fully reliable in identifying the eloquent structures, especially in cases where they are infiltrated by a glioma [65–68]. Therefore, when gliomas grow within or adjacent to eloquent regions, intraoperative electrophysiological monitoring of integrity and function of these structures is mandatory.

Direct electrical stimulation during AR of gliomas is currently considered to be the gold standard for the identification and preservation of language pathways [69]; this methodology is effective also in cases when functional pathways infiltrated by glioma cannot be displayed by tractography [65]. Direct electrical stimulation during AR is also a useful form of brain mapping of the language cortex [52], motor cortex and pathways [44, 70], visual cortex and pathways [40, 71, 72], etc.

Despite the fact that eloquent cortical and subcortical structures can be reliably identified by direct electrical stimulation and preserved during awake surgeries, this method is not able to identify glioma tissue. Therefore, like in the surgeries performed under general anesthesia, conventional neuronavigation and/or 2D-ultrasound is used in many centers during AR in order to local-

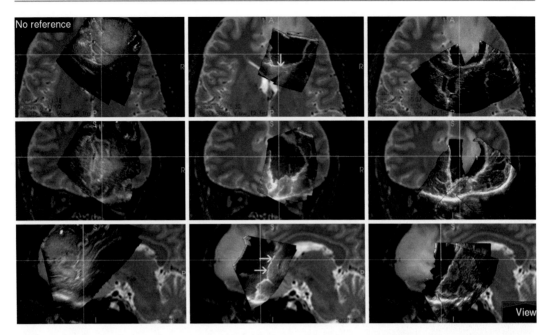

Fig. 8.5 Right-sided frontal grade II astrocytoma. *Left column*: Initial 3D-ultrasound image scanned from the dural surface fused with the preoperative navigation MRI showing a right-sided frontal grade II astrocytoma. *Middle column*: 3D-ultrasound scan performed from the dural surface during the resection. Note the hyperintensity at the bottom of the resection cavity; *yellow arrows,* corpus callosum and *red arrows*, inferior part of the right frontal lobe. Because these structures were not infiltrated (see initial 3D-ultrasound scan), the hyperintensity should be evaluated as the AEAs and not as a tumor remnant. *Right column*: AEAs were minimized by 3D-ultrasound data acquisition with a miniature probe inserted into the resection cavity; no hyperintense residual tumor is present at the bottom of the resection cavity. Surgery performed at the Department of Neurosurgery in Bratislava

ize glioma tissue [6–10, 52–56, 73]. Nevertheless, as mentioned before, the accuracy of neuronavigation is limited due to the brain-shift [28], and 2D-ultrasound is prone to image interpretation difficulties, especially after some tumor tissue debulking [43–45]. Due to these drawbacks, intraoperative MRI [30, 74–81] or navigated 3D-ultrasound [40, 49, 82] is used in several centers during AR of eloquently localized gliomas. Both methods enable distinct visualization of normal and pathological tissue, as well as intraoperative update of neuronavigation data and brain-shift compensation, which is critical for further course of the surgery.

The most prominent problem of AR is the limited time of the surgery due to patient fatigue [83]. Despite the described successful course of AR lasting up to 9 h [84], some patients can become tired within 1–2 h of resection [85]. In such cases, patients often demonstrate slowness in their language in the last stages of resection,

and it is not easy to differentiate language disturbances due to fatigue from the fact that the resection has interfered with language pathways [83].

Because the duration of AR is limited, intraoperative imaging modality used during these procedures should apart from distinct depiction of normal and pathological structures also allow fast update of navigation data. In this regard, 3D-ultrasound represents a very well-balanced intraoperative imaging modality. In addition to high-quality visualization of brain and tumor tissue, intraoperative data update may be repeatedly performed during the whole course of AR. Usually, the 3D-ultrasound navigation data update takes only 2–3 min [61], and therefore, the prolongation of the surgery is acceptable even in cases when several navigation data updates are needed.

Another important benefit of 3D-ultrasound is the possibility of intraoperative 3D visualization of normal and pathological vessels by power Doppler. According to the experiences gained

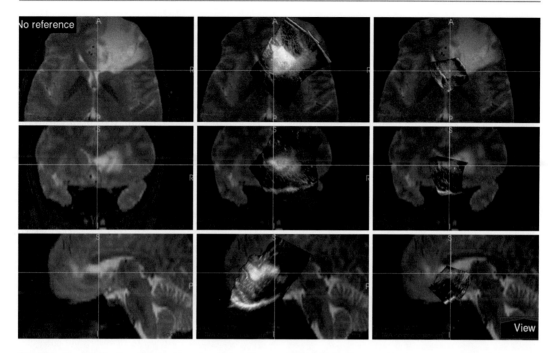

Fig. 8.6 3D visualization of tumor remnant. *Left column*: Preoperative 3D T2 MRI navigation sequence showing a right-sided frontal grade II oligoastrocytoma. *Middle column*: Initial 3D-ultrasound image scanned from the dural surface fused with the preoperative navigation MRI. *Right column*: 3D-ultrasound image acquired via scanning with mini-probe inserted within the resection cavity; the AEAs were minimized. Center of the yellow cross: tumor remnant in the corpus callosum. Surgery performed at the Department of Neurosurgery in Bratislava

during AR of insular gliomas performed in the Department of Neurosurgery in Bratislava, even lenticulostriate arteries may be visualized by navigated 3D-ultrasound (SonoWand Invite, SONOWAND AS, Trondheim, Norway) – unpublished data. Surprisingly, we were not able to find similar observation in the literature. Nevertheless, intraoperative visualization of lenticulostriate arteries (Fig. 8.7) and evaluation of the distance between these perforators and the bottom of the resection cavity during removal of insular gliomas (Fig. 8.8) may be of fundamental importance as injury to these vessels usually results in a dense hemiplegia [44]. On the other hand, reliability of lenticulostriate artery visualization by power Doppler is uncertain; a prospective study of this topic is needed. The future use of ultrasound contrast agents could probably contribute to even better lenticulostriate artery visualization.

A potential challenge before/during 3D-ultrasound-guided AR may be the positioning of the patient. During scanning the operating field with the ultrasound probe placed on the brain surface, the resection cavity has to be filled with saline [38]. If air becomes trapped in the resection cavity, the adequate visualization is usually compromised (Fig. 8.9). Therefore, the patient should be positioned so that the craniotomy plane is horizontal; in that way, saline will stay in the resection cavity. However, horizontal placement of the craniotomy in awake patients may be in some tumor locations difficult (e.g., in tumors growing close to the Rolandic area), as the patients' position during AR has to be comfortable. In the Department of Neurosurgery in Bratislava, a "miniature dam" made from bone wax is usually used, in order to keep the saline within the resection cavity in cases when the craniotomy is not placed horizontally (Fig. 8.10). Another possible solution in cases with nonhorizontal placement of the craniotomy is insertion of the hockey stick-shaped probe into the resection cavity [37].

8.2.4 Fluorescent Agents in Glioma Surgery, Combination with Intraoperative Ultrasound

Several authors have documented the use of sodium fluorescein during malignant glioma surgery, which has led to an increased number of complete resections [86, 87]. However, the data regarding the use of sodium fluorescein are still sparse. Another drug allowing fluorescence-based intraoperative identification of tumor tissue, 5-aminolevulinic acid (5-ALA), is used much more often.

Preoperative application of the 5-ALA leads to a preferential accumulation of its fluorescent metabolite, protoporphyrin IX, in malignant glioma cells. When illuminated under a blue light of wavelength $\lambda = 400–410$ nm, the protoporphyrin IX in the tumor glows an intense red, while the normal brain tissue appears blue [88]. The original use of 5-ALA was in the intraoperative identification and resection of contrast-enhancing malignant gliomas [88, 89]. Resections guided

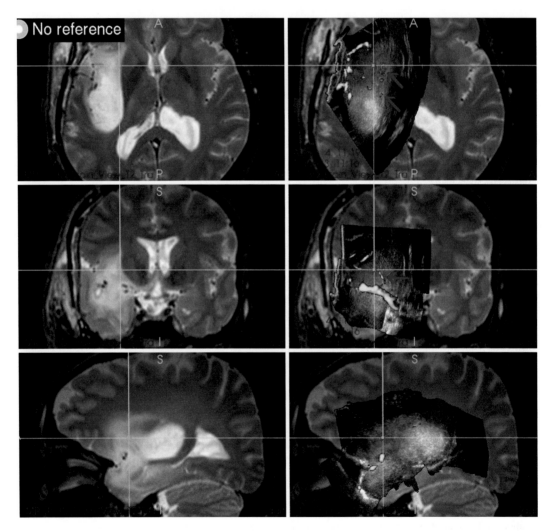

Fig. 8.7 Left-sided insular grade II astrocytoma. *Left column*: Preoperative 3D T2 MRI navigation sequence. *Right column*: 3D-ultrasound image acquired with 12 MHz linear probe fused with navigation MRI. Lenticulostriate arteries are clearly depicted by power Doppler (*red arrows*). Surgery performed at the Department of Neurosurgery in Bratislava

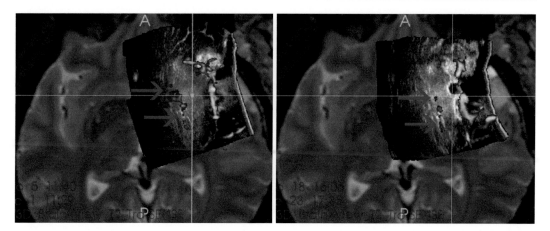

Fig. 8.8 Intraoperative visualization of lenticulostriate arteries (*arrows*) during AR of a right-sided insular grade II astrocytoma. *Left*: Intraoperative view after the beginning of resection. *Right*: Intraoperative view during the resection. Note that this allows the evaluation of the distance between lenticulostriate arteries and bottom of the resection cavity. Surgery performed at the Department of Neurosurgery in Bratislava

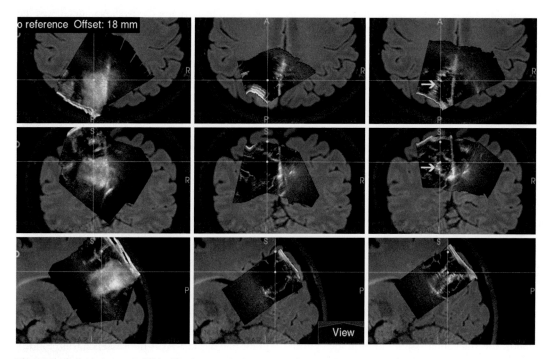

Fig. 8.9 *Left column*: Initial 3D-ultrasound image scanned from the dural surface fused with the navigation MRI showing a left-sided parietal grade II astrocytoma. *Middle column*: 3D-ultrasound scan performed from the dural surface after the resection. Note inadequate visualization of the resection cavity due to the trapped air – the position of the craniotomy was not horizontal. *Right column*: Adequate visualization of the resection cavity after using "miniature dam" made from bone wax, which allowed complete filling of the cavity with saline. A gross-total resection was achieved. *Arrow*: lateral border of the resection cavity. Surgery performed at the Department of Neurosurgery in Bratislava

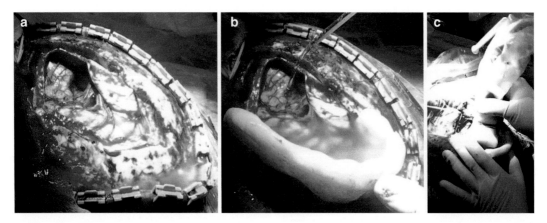

Fig. 8.10 Awake resection of a precentral glioma in a patient in semi-sitting position. (**a**) Complete filling of the resection cavity with saline was impossible as the craniotomy was not placed horizontally. (**b**) "Miniature dam" made from bone wax used in order to keep the saline within the resection cavity. (**c**) Subsequent intraoperative 3D-ultrasound data update. Surgery performed at the Department of Neurosurgery in Bratislava

by intraoperative 5-ALA usage were proven to be more radical as compared to resections without 5-ALA; in addition, the time to the tumor progression was longer when the resection was guided by 5-ALA [89]. A significant limit of the intraoperative 5-ALA use is the fact that even a thin layer of intervening, non-pathological tissue is enough to lead to incorrect impression of complete tumor resection [90, 91]. Heterogeneous tumors with low-grade parts and satellite malignant lesions cannot be reliably resected by fluorescence-guided surgery alone; in these cases, the additional use of intraoperative imaging is required [92–94].

Considering the fact that ultrasound is not able to selectively depict the contrast enhancing, i.e., most malignant part of high-grade gliomas (Fig. 8.11), the combination use with 5-ALA that is capable of selective malignant tissue visualization may be especially beneficial. On the other hand, the fact that some high-grade glioma patients may benefit from further resection of T2 abnormality [95] that can be visualized by ultra-

sound but usually not by 5-ALA underscores the potential benefit of combining these methods. Another potential technique to differentiate between malignant glioma tissue and peritumoral edema is application of ultrasound contrast agents [96]; however, future prospective studies are necessary to confirm the efficacy of this method.

In 2010, Widhalm et al. described a new intraoperative utilization of 5-ALA fluorescence [97]. The authors used 5-ALA in order to serve as a marker for direct intraoperative detection of anaplastic foci within infiltrative supratentorial gliomas with no or nonsignificant contrast enhancement. Anaplastic glioma foci could be discerned as red-fluorescing spots during illumination of operating field with violet-blue light. One of the most important advantages of this method is the fact that it is unaffected by brainshift [97]. A good correlation between tumor grade and tissue 5-ALA fluorescence was reported later by Steno et al. [98] and in an update of the pilot series reported by Widhalm et al. [99].

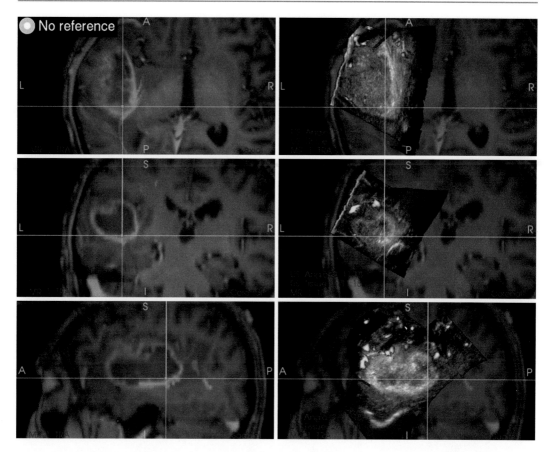

Fig. 8.11 Left-sided temporal glioblastoma surrounded by edema. *Left column*: Preoperative contrast-enhanced 3D T1 MRI navigation sequence. *Right column*: 3D-ultrasound image fused with navigation MRI. Contrast-enhancing malignant tissue is better distinguishable by MRI; both tumor tissue and peritumoral edema are hyperechoic on ultrasound image. Surgery performed at the Department of Neurosurgery in Bratislava

Regarding the latter 5-ALA utilization, again, concurrent intraoperative use of 5-ALA and 3D-ultrasound may represent additional benefit. In focally malignized low-grade gliomas, the goal of the surgery is an extensive resection and identification of the anaplastic foci in order to avoid sampling error. In such cases, 3D-ultrasound provides adequate visualization of the whole hyperechogenic tumor, while the anaplastic foci can be intraoperatively identified by 5-ALA fluorescence (Fig. 8.12).

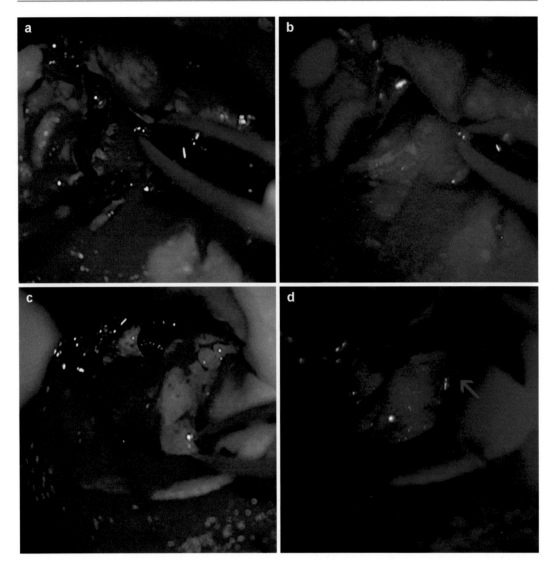

Fig. 8.12 Resection of right-sided insular astrocytoma (MRI and 3D-ultrasound image were shown in Fig. 8.3). (**a**) Tumor removal via transsylvian approach. (**b**) Repeated illumination of the operating field revealed no fluorescence in vast majority of the tumor tissue. All non-fluorescing tissue was postoperatively histopathologically evaluated as grade II (**c**) partially resected deep subcortical tumor portion (pulled out to the brain surface). (**d**) Solitary minute 5-ALA-positive focus (postoperatively histopathologically evaluated as high-grade glioma) was found in this tumor part (*red arrow*). Surgery performed at the Department of Neurosurgery in Bratislava

References

1. Jakola AS et al (2012) Comparison of a strategy favoring early surgical resection vs a strategy favoring watchful waiting in low-grade gliomas. JAMA 308(18):1881–1888
2. Eyupoglu IY, Buchfelder M, Savaskan NE (2013) Surgical resection of malignant gliomas-role in optimizing patient outcome. Nat Rev Neurol 9(3):141–151
3. Perry A (2003) Pathology of low-grade gliomas: an update of emerging concepts. Neuro Oncol 5(3):168–178
4. Wirtz CR et al (2000) The benefit of neuronavigation for neurosurgery analyzed by its impact on glioblastoma surgery. Neurol Res 22(4):354–360
5. Kurimoto M et al (2004) Impact of neuronavigation and image-guided extensive resection for adult patients with supratentorial malignant astrocytomas: a single-institution retrospective study. Minim Invasive Neurosurg 47(5):278–283

6. Bello L et al (2007) Intraoperative subcortical language tract mapping guides surgical removal of gliomas involving speech areas. Neurosurgery 60(1):67–80; discussion 80–82
7. Mert A et al (2015) Introduction of a standardized multimodality image protocol for navigation-guided surgery of suspected low-grade gliomas. Neurosurg Focus 38(1):E4
8. Leuthardt EC et al (2002) Frameless stereotaxy without rigid pin fixation during awake craniotomies. Stereotact Funct Neurosurg 79(3–4):256–261
9. Pinsker MO, Nabavi A, Mehdorn HM (2007) Neuronavigation and resection of lesions located in eloquent brain areas under local anesthesia and neuropsychological-neurophysiological monitoring. Minim Invasive Neurosurg 50(5):281–284
10. Chang EF et al (2008) Preoperative prognostic classification system for hemispheric low-grade gliomas in adults. J Neurosurg 109(5):817–824
11. Willems PW et al (2006) Effectiveness of neuronavigation in resecting solitary intracerebral contrast-enhancing tumors: a randomized controlled trial. J Neurosurg 104(3):360–368
12. Nimsky C (2011) Intraoperative MRI in glioma surgery: proof of benefit? Lancet Oncol 12(11):982–983
13. Knauth M et al (1999) Intraoperative MR imaging increases the extent of tumor resection in patients with high-grade gliomas. AJNR Am J Neuroradiol 20(9):1642–1646
14. Wirtz CR et al (2000) Clinical evaluation and follow-up results for intraoperative magnetic resonance imaging in neurosurgery. Neurosurgery 46(5):1112–1120; discussion 1120–1122
15. Bohinski RJ et al (2001) Glioma resection in a shared-resource magnetic resonance operating room after optimal image-guided frameless stereotactic resection. Neurosurgery 48(4):731–742; discussion 742–744
16. Nimsky C et al (2003) Glioma surgery evaluated by intraoperative low-field magnetic resonance imaging. Acta Neurochir Suppl 85:55–63
17. Hirschberg H et al (2005) Impact of intraoperative MRI on the surgical results for high-grade gliomas. Minim Invasive Neurosurg 48(2):77–84
18. Schneider JP et al (2005) Intraoperative MRI to guide the resection of primary supratentorial glioblastoma multiforme--a quantitative radiological analysis. Neuroradiology 47(7):489–500
19. Hatiboglu MA et al (2010) Utilization of intraoperative motor mapping in glioma surgery with high-field intraoperative magnetic resonance imaging. Stereotact Funct Neurosurg 88(6):345–352
20. Pamir MN et al (2010) First intraoperative, shared-resource, ultrahigh-field 3-Tesla magnetic resonance imaging system and its application in low-grade glioma resection. J Neurosurg 112(1):57–69
21. Senft C et al (2011) Intraoperative MRI guidance and extent of resection in glioma surgery: a randomised, controlled trial. Lancet Oncol 12(11):997–1003
22. Kubben PL et al (2011) Intraoperative MRI-guided resection of glioblastoma multiforme: a systematic review. Lancet Oncol 12(11):1062–1070
23. Barone DG, Lawrie TA, Hart MG (2014) Image guided surgery for the resection of brain tumours. Cochrane Database Syst Rev 1:Cd009685
24. Nimsky C et al (2005) Preoperative and intraoperative diffusion tensor imaging-based fiber tracking in glioma surgery. Neurosurgery 56(1):130–137; discussion 138
25. Seifert V, Gasser T, Senft C (2011) Low field intraoperative MRI in glioma surgery. Acta Neurochir Suppl 109:35–41
26. Bellut D et al (2010) Intraoperative magnetic resonance imaging-assisted transsphenoidal pituitary surgery in patients with acromegaly. Neurosurg Focus 29(4):E9
27. Moiyadi A, Shetty P (2011) Objective assessment of utility of intraoperative ultrasound in resection of central nervous system tumors: a cost-effective tool for intraoperative navigation in neurosurgery. J Neurosci Rural Pract 2(1):4–11
28. Nimsky C, Ganslandt O, Fahlbusch R (2006) Implementation of fiber tract navigation. Neurosurgery 58(4 Suppl 2):ONS-292–ONS-303; discussion ONS-303-ONS-304
29. Ostry S et al (2013) Is intraoperative diffusion tensor imaging at 3.0T comparable to subcortical corticospinal tract mapping? Neurosurgery 73(5):797–807; discussion 806–807
30. Peruzzi P et al (2011) Intraoperative MRI (ioMRI) in the setting of awake craniotomies for supratentorial glioma resection. Acta Neurochir Suppl 109:43–48
31. Rubin JM et al (1980) Intraoperative ultrasound examination of the brain. Radiology 137(3):831–832
32. Sosna J et al (2005) Intraoperative sonography for neurosurgery. J Ultrasound Med 24(12):1671–1682
33. Nimsky C, Carl B (2015) Intraoperative imaging. In: Golby AJ (ed) Image-guided neurosurgery. Elsevier, San Diego/Waltham/Oxford, pp 163–190
34. Unsgaard G et al (2002) Brain operations guided by real-time two-dimensional ultrasound: new possibilities as a result of improved image quality. Neurosurgery 51(2):402–411; discussion 411–412
35. Unsgaard G et al (2006) Intra-operative 3D ultrasound in neurosurgery. Acta Neurochir (Wien) 148(3):235–253; discussion 253
36. Coburger J et al (2014) Navigated high frequency ultrasound: description of technique and clinical comparison with conventional intracranial ultrasound. World Neurosurg 82(3–4):366–375
37. Coburger J et al (2015) Linear array ultrasound in low-grade glioma surgery: histology-based assessment of accuracy in comparison to conventional intraoperative ultrasound and intraoperative MRI. Acta Neurochir (Wien) 157(2):195–206
38. Unsgard G et al (2011) Intra-operative imaging with 3D ultrasound in neurosurgery. Acta Neurochir Suppl 109:181–186

39. Unsgaard G et al (2005) Ability of navigated 3D ultrasound to delineate gliomas and metastases – comparison of image interpretations with histopathology. Acta Neurochir (Wien) 147(12):1259–1269; discussion 1269

40. Steno A et al (2012) Navigated three-dimensional intraoperative ultrasound-guided awake resection of low-grade glioma partially infiltrating optic radiation. Acta Neurochir (Wien) 154(7):1255–1262

41. Moiyadi AV et al (2013) Usefulness of three-dimensional navigable intraoperative ultrasound in resection of brain tumors with a special emphasis on malignant gliomas. Acta Neurochir (Wien) 155(12):2217–2225

42. Solheim O et al (2010) Ultrasound-guided operations in unselected high-grade gliomas – overall results, impact of image quality and patient selection. Acta Neurochir (Wien) 152(11):1873–1886

43. Petridis AK et al (2015) The value of intraoperative sonography in low grade glioma surgery. Clin Neurol Neurosurg 131:64–68

44. Hentschel SJ, Lang FF (2005) Surgical resection of intrinsic insular tumors. Neurosurgery 57(1 Suppl):176–183; discussion 176–183

45. Gerganov VM et al (2011) Two-dimensional high-end ultrasound imaging compared to intraoperative MRI during resection of low-grade gliomas. J Clin Neurosci 18(5):669–673

46. Selbekk T et al (2013) Ultrasound imaging in neurosurgery: approaches to minimize surgically induced image artefacts for improved resection control. Acta Neurochir (Wien) 155(6):973–980

47. Jakola AS et al (2014) Animal study assessing safety of an acoustic coupling fluid that holds the potential to avoid surgically induced artifacts in 3D ultrasound guided operations. BMC Med Imaging 14:11

48. Steno A, Matejcik V, Steno J (2015) Intraoperative ultrasound in low-grade glioma surgery. Clin Neurol Neurosurg 135:96–99

49. Steno A et al (2014) Direct electrical stimulation of the optic radiation in patients with covered eyes. Neurosurg Rev 37(3):527–533; discussion 533

50. Bozinov O et al (2011) Advantages and limitations of intraoperative 3D ultrasound in neurosurgery. Technical note. Acta Neurochir Suppl 109:191–196

51. Unsgaard G et al (2002) Neuronavigation by intraoperative three-dimensional ultrasound: initial experience during brain tumor resection. Neurosurgery 50(4):804–812; discussion 812

52. Duffau H et al (2008) Intraoperative subcortical stimulation mapping of language pathways in a consecutive series of 115 patients with Grade II glioma in the left dominant hemisphere. J Neurosurg 109(3):461–471

53. Bai HM et al (2011) Three core techniques in surgery of neuroepithelial tumors in eloquent areas: awake anaesthesia, intraoperative direct electrical stimulation and ultrasonography. Chin Med J (Engl) 124(19):3035–3041

54. Kim SS et al (2009) Awake craniotomy for brain tumors near eloquent cortex: correlation of intraoperative cortical mapping with neurological outcomes in 309 consecutive patients. Neurosurgery 64(5):836–845; discussion 345–346

55. Chacko AG et al (2013) Awake craniotomy and electrophysiological mapping for eloquent area tumours. Clin Neurol Neurosurg 115(3):329–334

56. Zhang Z et al (2008) Surgical strategies for glioma involving language areas. Chin Med J (Engl) 121(18):1800–1805

57. Prada F et al (2014) Intraoperative contrast-enhanced ultrasound for brain tumor surgery. Neurosurgery 74(5):542–552; discussion 552

58. Hata N et al (1997) Development of a frameless and armless stereotactic neuronavigation system with ultrasonographic registration. Neurosurgery 41(3):608–613; discussion 613–614

59. Koivukangas J et al (1993) Ultrasound-controlled neuronavigator-guided brain surgery. J Neurosurg 79(1):36–42

60. Trobaugh JW et al (1994) Frameless stereotactic ultrasonography: method and applications. Comput Med Imaging Graph 18(4):235–246

61. Gronningsaeter A et al (2000) SonoWand, an ultrasound-based neuronavigation system. Neurosurgery 47(6):1373–1379; discussion 1379–1380

62. Lindseth F et al (2003) Multimodal image fusion in ultrasound-based neuronavigation: improving overview and interpretation by integrating preoperative MRI with intraoperative 3D ultrasound. Comput Aided Surg 8(2):49–69

63. Skirboll SS et al (1996) Functional cortex and subcortical white matter located within gliomas. Neurosurgery 38(4):678–684; discussion 684–685

64. Schiffbauer H et al (2001) Functional activity within brain tumors: a magnetic source imaging study. Neurosurgery 49(6):1313–1320; discussion 1320–1321

65. Leclercq D et al (2010) Comparison of diffusion tensor imaging tractography of language tracts and intraoperative subcortical stimulations. J Neurosurg 112(3):503–511

66. Giussani C et al (2010) Is preoperative functional magnetic resonance imaging reliable for language areas mapping in brain tumor surgery? Review of language functional magnetic resonance imaging and direct cortical stimulation correlation studies. Neurosurgery 66(1):113–120

67. Wilden JA et al (2013) Strategies to maximize resection of complex, or high surgical risk, low-grade gliomas. Neurosurg Focus 34(2):E5

68. Mandelli ML et al (2014) Quantifying accuracy and precision of diffusion MR tractography of the corticospinal tract in brain tumors. J Neurosurg 121(2):349–358

69. Sanai N, Chang S, Berger MS (2011) Low-grade gliomas in adults. J Neurosurg 115(5):948–965

70. Fontaine D, Capelle L, Duffau H (2002) Somatotopy of the supplementary motor area: evidence from correlation of the extent of surgical resection with the clinical patterns of deficit. Neurosurgery 50(2):297–303; discussion 303–305

71. Nguyen HS et al (2011) A method to map the visual cortex during an awake craniotomy. J Neurosurg 114(4):922–926

72. Gras-Combe G et al (2012) Intraoperative subcortical electrical mapping of optic radiations in awake surgery for glioma involving visual pathways. J Neurosurg 117(3):466–473

73. Berger MS, Hadjipanayis CG (2007) Surgery of intrinsic cerebral tumors. Neurosurgery 61(1 Suppl):279–304; discussion 304–305

74. Maldaun MV et al (2014) Awake craniotomy for gliomas in a high-field intraoperative magnetic resonance imaging suite: analysis of 42 cases. J Neurosurg 121(4):810–817

75. Goebel S et al (2010) Patient perception of combined awake brain tumor surgery and intraoperative 1.5-T magnetic resonance imaging: the Kiel experience. Neurosurgery 67(3):594–600; discussion 600

76. Leuthardt EC et al (2011) Use of movable high-field-strength intraoperative magnetic resonance imaging with awake craniotomies for resection of gliomas: preliminary experience. Neurosurgery 69(1):194–205; discussion 205–206

77. Lu J et al (2013) Awake language mapping and 3-Tesla intraoperative MRI-guided volumetric resection for gliomas in language areas. J Clin Neurosci 20(9):1280–1287

78. Parney IF et al (2010) Awake craniotomy, electrophysiologic mapping, and tumor resection with high-field intraoperative MRI. World Neurosurg 73(5):547–551

79. Tuominen J et al (2013) Awake craniotomy may further improve neurological outcome of intraoperative MRI-guided brain tumor surgery. Acta Neurochir (Wien) 155(10):1805–1812

80. Takrouri MS et al (2010) Conscious sedation for awake craniotomy in intraoperative magnetic resonance imaging operating theater. Anesth Essays Res 4(1):33–37

81. Nabavi A et al (2009) Awake craniotomy and intraoperative magnetic resonance imaging: patient selection, preparation, and technique. Top Magn Reson Imaging 19(4):191–196

82. Nossek E et al (2011) Intraoperative mapping and monitoring of the corticospinal tracts with neurophysiological assessment and 3-dimensional ultrasonography-based navigation. Clinical article. J Neurosurg 114(3):738–746

83. Duffau H et al (2003) Usefulness of intraoperative electrical subcortical mapping during surgery for low-grade gliomas located within eloquent brain regions: functional results in a consecutive series of 103 patients. J Neurosurg 98(4):764–778

84. Garavaglia MM et al (2014) Anesthetic approach to high-risk patients and prolonged awake craniotomy using dexmedetomidine and scalp block. J Neurosurg Anesthesiol 26(3):226–233

85. Duffau H (2013) Surgery for diffuse Low-grade gliomas (DLGG) functional considerations. In: Duffau H (ed) Diffuse low-grade gliomas in adults. Springer, London, pp 375–399

86. Koc K et al (2008) Fluorescein sodium-guided surgery in glioblastoma multiforme: a prospective evaluation. Br J Neurosurg 22(1):99–103

87. Shinoda J et al (2003) Fluorescence-guided resection of glioblastoma multiforme by using high-dose fluorescein sodium. Technical note. J Neurosurg 99(3):597–603

88. Stummer W et al (1998) Intraoperative detection of malignant gliomas by 5-aminolevulinic acid-induced porphyrin fluorescence. Neurosurgery 42(3):518–525; discussion 525–526

89. Stummer W et al (2006) Fluorescence-guided surgery with 5-aminolevulinic acid for resection of malignant glioma: a randomised controlled multicentre phase III trial. Lancet Oncol 7(5):392–401

90. Feigl GC et al (2010) Resection of malignant brain tumors in eloquent cortical areas: a new multimodal approach combining 5-aminolevulinic acid and intraoperative monitoring. J Neurosurg 113(2):352–357

91. Eyupoglu IY et al (2012) Improving the extent of malignant glioma resection by dual intraoperative visualization approach. PLoS One 7(9):e44885

92. Hefti M et al (2008) 5-aminolevulinic acid induced protoporphyrin IX fluorescence in high-grade glioma surgery: a one-year experience at a single institution. Swiss Med Wkly 138(11–12):180–185

93. Tsugu A et al (2011) Impact of the combination of 5-aminolevulinic acid-induced fluorescence with intraoperative magnetic resonance imaging-guided surgery for glioma. World Neurosurg 76(1–2):120–127

94. Moiyadi A, Shetty P (2014) Navigable intraoperative ultrasound and fluorescence-guided resections are complementary in resection control of malignant gliomas: one size does not fit all. J Neurol Surg A Cent Eur Neurosurg 75(6):434–441

95. Beiko J et al (2014) IDH1 mutant malignant astrocytomas are more amenable to surgical resection and have a survival benefit associated with maximal surgical resection. Neuro Oncol 16(1):81–91

96. Prada F et al (2014) Intraoperative cerebral glioma characterization with contrast enhanced ultrasound. Biomed Res Int 2014:1–9

97. Widhalm G et al (2010) 5-Aminolevulinic acid is a promising marker for detection of anaplastic foci in diffusely infiltrating gliomas with nonsignificant contrast enhancement. Cancer 116(6):1545–1552

98. Steno A et al (2012) Detection of anaplastic foci within infiltrative gliomas with nonsignificant contrast enhancement using 5-aminolevulic acid – a report of five cases. Cesk Slov Neurol 75(108):227–232

99. Widhalm G et al (2013) 5-Aminolevulinic acid induced fluorescence is a powerful intraoperative marker for precise histopathological grading of gliomas with non-significant contrast-enhancement. PLoS One 8(10):e76988

Part III

Doppler Imaging

Doppler Imaging: Basic Principles and Clinical Application

9

Valentina Caldiera, Luigi Caputi, and Elisa Ciceri

9.1 Introduction

The echo-color Doppler technique [1–4] includes:

1. Echo: B-mode technique represents the anatomical background as a bidimensional image in scale of grey.
2. Color flow: Dynamic colorimetric imaging superimposed to the anatomical background encoding velocities and flow direction.
3. Spectral Doppler: Gives information on velocities and direction of the flux in a selected vessel. It enables to obtain a spectrum of flow velocities over time.

9.1.1 Probes

In the most of neurological studies, linear transducers with frequencies of 7–10 MHz are utilized to study superficial vessels located at a depth of 2–4 cm; lower frequencies with conventional convex probes, instead, are requested to investi-

V. Caldiera, MD (✉) • E. Ciceri, MD
Neuroradiology Unit, Fondazione IRCCS Istituto
Neurologico C. Besta, via Celoria 11,
Milan 20133, Italy
e-mail: valentina.caldiera@istituto-besta.it

L. Caputi, MD
Department of Cerebrovascular Diseases, Fondazione
IRCCS Istituto Neurologico C. Besta, Milan, Italy

gate deep vasculature up to a depth of 20–25 cm from the skin. In neurosurgery, a linear array multifrequency (3–11 MHz) probe with trapezoidal view is usually utilized for the examination.

9.1.2 Anatomical Background and Depiction of the Vessels

Morphological images are depicted according to B-mode technique. Vessels of interest must be explored along both the axial and the longitudinal planes (Fig. 9.1), in order to depict plaques or arterial thickenings.

Imaging can be improved by regulating the probe frequency, the depth and the field of view, and the total gain, as seen in the previous chapters. In order to obtain a good visualization of the anatomical background, the studied vessel must be homogeneously insonated.

9.1.3 Doppler Imaging: Physical Principles

After the morphological evaluation, flow analysis can be applied by Doppler technique.

Colorimetric imaging and Doppler spectra are both extracted by the Doppler equation that represents the so-called Doppler effect; this is a physic phenomenon where by a radiofrequency

© Springer International Publishing Switzerland 2016
F. Prada et al. (eds.), *Intraoperative Ultrasound (IOUS) in Neurosurgery:*
From Standard B-mode to Elastosonography, DOI 10.1007/978-3-319-25268-1_9

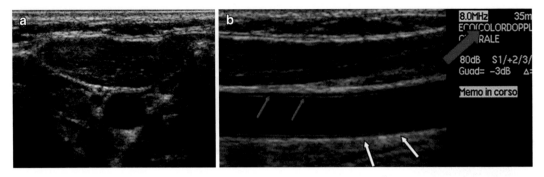

Fig. 9.1 Echo B-mode of the common carotid artery. The vessel is explored along both transverse (**a**) and axial plane (**b**). Parameters must be set in order to obtain the complete insonation of the vessel. Examination is per- formed with a linear probe of 8 MHz (*red arrow*). Note the good visualization of the intima (*pink arrows*) and adventitia layers (*white arrows*)

(RF) wave that vibrates at a specific frequency changes vibration rate when reflecting on a moving surface (red blood cells, for instance) according to the following formula:

$$\Delta F = \frac{2F_i v \cos \theta}{c}$$

where ΔF is the depicted (reflexed) radiofrequency, F_i the incident RF wave, v the velocity of the moving surface, θ the angle of incidence between the incident wave and the moving surface, and c the velocity of ultrasound (US) in the tissue. The depicted wave is directly proportional to the *velocity of the blood,* which could be extracted from the previous equation as

$$v = \frac{\Delta F c}{2F_i v \cos \theta}$$

Therefore, Doppler signal and color Doppler are proportional to the *incidence angle* (IA) between the incident wave and the moving surface (Fig. 9.2a, b). Thus, in order to obtain a depicted velocity close to the real one, the probe must be as much parallel as possible to the moving blood cells (cosine 0° = 1). Perpendicular angles (cosine 90° = 0) between incident wave and moving surface will cause cancellation or weakening of the signal received (Fig. 9.2c).

The best incidence angle to obtain a good imaging is different between B-mode and Doppler imaging. The former technique obtains better information utilizing an IA angle close to 90°(perpendicular to the vessel), whereas the latter one utilizing an IA angle parallel to the long axis of the studied vessel requires angles as much close to 0° as possible. Angles between 30° and 60° represent a good compromise in standard clinical practice.

Doppler imaging can be performed with continuous wave or pulsed wave Doppler system. The continuous Doppler system utilizes an ultrasound (US) probe that is equipped with two piezoelectric crystals, a continuous RF wave producer, and a distinct RF receiver, for detection of the returning waves. There are no limitations to the range velocities that could be explored with this technique. However, this examination enables to study only the velocity curve distribution inside the vessels, without offering any associate morphological information. Also, the exact location of the detected signals cannot be defined because all the returning RT waves, reflected by the whole tissue, are recorded. Instead, pulsed Doppler technique utilizes a US probe where the same piezoelectric crystal alternately works as emitting and receiving device. In this case, time length and rhythm of emitted/received waves can be regulated with an electronic window that enables to select dimensions and position of the explored area (color box, Fig. 9.2). Frequency of transmission is called *pulse repetition frequency* (PRF) and, in most of the existing equipment, is coupled with the maximum displayed velocity in the *velocity scale*

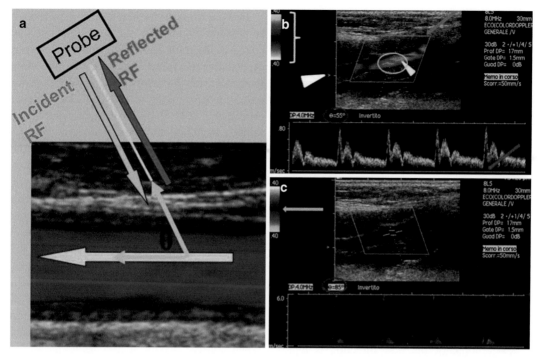

Fig. 9.2 (**a**) Graphical representation of Doppler effect. θ is the angle comprised between radiofrequencies (*RF*) coming from/directed to the probe (*green* and *blue arrows*) and the direction of blood flow (*yellow arrow*). In (**b**, **c**) an example of Doppler signal angle dependency is shown. (**b**) Doppler imaging obtained with an angle of 55° (*red circle*) shows a good Doppler signal represented as a homogeneous color filling of the vessel and a correspon-dent good spectral analysis. (**c**) The same scan obtained with an angle of 85° (*red circle*) shows cancellation of the signal in the color box and a poor spectrum with aliasing. *Yellow brace*: color scale (velocity scale of color flow). *White arrowhead*: focus. *Pink arrow*: color baseline. *Purple arrow*: color box. *Red arrow*: spectral baseline. *Green circle*: sample volume of spectral Doppler. *Yellow arrowhead: cursor*

that defines the limit of the detectable velocity (Fig. 9.2). The repetition interval is determined by the total time that the impulse requires to reach the selected area and to return to the receiver. An important limitation of pulsed Doppler is the incapability to correctly detect velocities higher than one-half PRF (Nyquist limit), resulting in a misinterpretation of the Doppler signal known as *aliasing* phenomenon. In fact, the time interval between sampling pulses must be sufficient for a pulse to make the return journey from the transducer to the reflector and back. If a second pulse is sent before the first is received, the receiver cannot discriminate between the reflected signals from both pulses, and ambiguity ensues in the range of the sample volume. As the depth of investigation increases, the pulse journey time to and from the reflector increases and it becomes necessary to reduce the *PRF* in order to maintain an unambiguu-

ous velocity ranging, so as to avoid an aliasing effect. Therefore, utilizing this technique, the maximum measurable frequency decreases with the depth. However, low pulse repetition frequencies can be useful to examine low-velocity vessels (e.g., venous flow). The longer interval between pulses allows the scanner a greater chance of identifying slow flow. However, the aliasing effect can also occur while low *PRF* or velocity scales are used, when high flow velocities are encountered. Conversely, if a high pulse repetition frequency is used to examine high velocities, low velocities may not be identified.

9.1.4   Color Flow Imaging

A color box (Fig. 9.2) can be superimposed on the anatomical background in order to obtain a colorimetric representation of the flow characteristics, direction, and velocity, in the selected area of interest. Size and location of the box can be manually regulated to cover the area of interest; increasing its size or width will result in a reduction of frame rate and in an increase of the required processing power and time. Thus, the overlay should be as small and superficial as possible.

A too large overlay reducing the frame rate will result in lower flow depiction. A too deep color box will result in slower PRF, which may produce aliasing in color flow map. Additionally, the focus parameter must be set at the region of interest in order to obtain a more accurate representation of flow (Fig. 9.2). The angle of incidence and the *PRF* will be set according to the anatomy region and the blood flow velocity, and the second one increased for faster fluxes and reduced in case of slow velocities, as already discussed.

Conventionally, the flow direction is represented in red if moving toward the probe (arterial flow) and in blue if moving away from the probe (venous flow). Velocities are encoded by color saturation, utilizing different shades of red and blue: conventionally, lighter shades of color are assigned to higher velocities. The color/velocity coupling is reported on the *color scale* (or *velocity scale*) (Fig. 9.2) where the scale of colors assigned to the different velocities and the limits of detectable velocities are displayed. A black line divides the color bar into positive or negative Doppler shifts; this line is called *color baseline* (Fig. 9.2). The color baseline can be adjusted to emphasize certain aspects of flow without changing the overall range of detectable velocities. For instance, by lowering the color baseline, the emphasis will be on flow directed toward the transducer; thus, the maximum velocity detectable in the positive side of the color scale will be higher, whereas the maximum velocity in the negative side will be reduced. This function can be used to correct aliasing in case of velocities exceeding the range comprised in the color scale; when aliasing occurs, the maximum detectable velocity in the direction of flow of the studied vessel can be increased by changing this parameter (Fig. 9.4).

In order to obtain the best flow visualization, it is possible to regulate the *gain* function that increases the color filling in the vessel. However, excessive *gain* values can produce false flow images outside the vessels or images of oversaturation, whereas low values can cause signal cancellation (Fig. 9.3). The correct color image setting, including the *gain* regulation, can be visually adjusted real-time by the operator at the console during the exam. In case of laminar flow, color image will display a parabolic distribution of velocity vectors through the vessel, with brighter colors at the center of the vessel (higher velocities) and darker colors closer to the vessel wall (slow velocities). In case of turbulences, the Doppler will demonstrate an inhomogeneous color map representing different directions and velocities concentrated in the same region of interest. *PRF* must be set according to blood velocities in order to avoid aliasing phenomena. When aliasing occurs, it appears as an abrupt shift of color from red to blue or vice versa in points of faster motion (Fig. 9.4a), as frequently observed in cases of vessel stenosis. The brightest shades of red and blue lie adjacent to each other at the aliasing point.

Practical guidelines are reported in Table 9.1.

9.1.5 Spectral Doppler

Pulsed wave Doppler ultrasound is used to provide a sonogram of the vessel (artery or vein) under investigation. It is performed by placing a small *sample volume* in the area of interest of the vessel on color images. The *sample volume* (Fig. 9.2) delimits an area comprised by two parallel lines, whose distance can be regulated. A cursor must be oriented according to flow direction (Fig. 9.2). The less volume studied, the more accurate the analysis. The best resolution of the sonogram occurs when the B-mode image and color image are frozen. If concurrent imaging is used (real-time duplex or triplex imaging), the temporal resolution of the sonogram is compromised.

Analogously to color Doppler, *PRF* (*velocity scale*) must be adjusted according to the blood velocities to avoid aliasing; when this eventuality

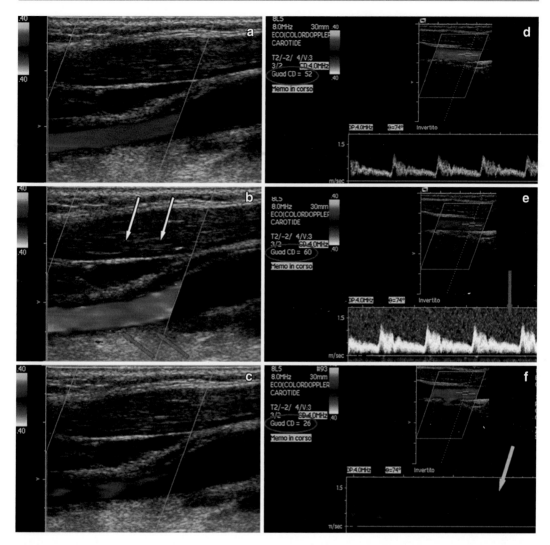

Fig. 9.3 Gain setting in color (**a–c**) and spectral (**d–f**) Doppler. (**a**) Optimal color gain with a good visualization of blood flow in the vessel. (**b**) Excessive increase in color gain values causes less shaped color filling in the vessel (*pink arrows*) and appearance of false flow images in the soft tissues (*white arrows*). (**c**) Low color gain values generate reduction in Doppler signal. (**d**) Optimal gain setting in spectral Doppler. (**e**) Excessive gain generates a noisy spectrum (*pink arrow*). (**f**) Low gain causes attenuation/cancellation of the spectrum (*green arrow*)

occurs, velocities exceeding the detecting capability are represented in the opposite side of the spectrum (Fig. 9.4). Like the color baseline, the *spectral baseline* (Fig. 9.2) can be altered to improve depiction of the spectral waveform (Fig. 9.4). This adjustment, which represents another way to prevent aliasing, allows the waveform to be brought down onto the baseline; even if it does not change the overall range of velocities that can be depicted, it increases the maximum detectable

velocity in the positive or negative side of the spectrum.

In addition, an adequate *gain* must be set to clearly visualize the spectrum free of noise (Fig. 9.3). Doppler imaging results in a spectral graph, which represents the speed changes of flow throughout the cardiac cycle and the distribution of the velocities that were recorded in the sample volume area. The spectrum of a normal laminar flow will show vectors in the higher part of the

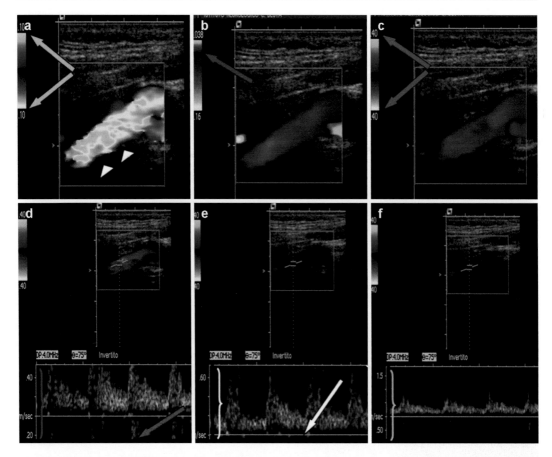

Fig. 9.4 Correction of aliasing by adjusting velocity scale or baseline during color flow (**a–c**) and spectral Doppler (**d–f**). (**a**) Aliasing phenomena are visible in the color box (*white arrowheads*). Green arrows show the color scale and the range of velocities that can be correctly detected, comprised between 0.10 and −0.10 m/s. (**b**) Adjustment of the baseline (*red arrow*) can correct aliasing without changing the overall range of velocities that can be depicted. (**c**) Adjustment of color scale values changes PRF and the range of velocities that can be depicted in both directions (*blue arrows*). (**d**) Aliasing phenomena in the spectral graph can be seen as an abrupt cut of the upper side of the spectrum; velocities exceeding the detecting capability are represented in the opposite side of the spectrum (*pink arrow*). (**e**) Lowering the baseline (*white arrow*, compare with (**d**)) can correct aliasing without changing the overall range of velocities (*white brace*). (**f**) Adjustment of velocity scale (*green brace*) values changes PRF and the range of velocities that can be depicted in both direction of flow

spectrum with frequencies near the highest frequencies, whether the area below the curve will be empty; instead, in the presence of a turbulent flow, a wide range of velocities will be detected; thus, also the lower part of the spectrum will be filled of vectors.

Many different indices have been used to describe the shape of flow waveform. All are designed to describe the waveform in a quantitative way. In general terms, they are a compromise between simplicity and the amount of information obtained. The indices that are commonly available on most commercial scanners are as follows:

1. Resistance index (RI) (also called resistive index or Pourcclot's index)
2. Systolic/diastolic (S/D) ratio, sometimes called the A/B ratio
3. Pulsatility index (PI)

Table 9.1 Suggested procedure to obtain a correct color flow imaging

Color flow imaging-practical guidelines
Ensure focus is at the region of interest. See Fig. 9.2
Set the color flow region to appropriate size. A smaller color box may lead to a better frame rate and better color resolution/sensitivity. See Fig. 9.2
Angle the probe or oblique color box (linear probes) to obtain an optimal beam-vessel angle (comprised between 30° and 60°). See Fig. 9.2
Adjust gain to obtain an appropriate imaging. See Fig. 9.3

Adapt PRF/velocity scale according to flow conditions and to avoid aliasing:
   Low PRF are more sensitive to low flows/velocities but may produce aliasing.
   High PRF are less sensitive to low velocities but reduce aliasing
 See Fig. 9.4

Adjust color baseline to avoid aliasing. See Fig. 9.4

Table 9.2 Suggested procedure in spectral Doppler analysis

Spectral Doppler-practical guidelines
Set the sample volume positioned on the vessel under investigation to correct size (small volumes enable to obtain a more accurate signal depiction. See Fig. 9.2
Oblique the cursor along the direction of blood flow. See Fig. 9.2
Oblique color box or position the probe to obtain an optimal beam-vessel angle (angles close to 90° will gave unclear values. Angles should be set to values <60°). See Fig. 9.2
Adjust gain to obtain a sonogram free of noise. See Fig. 9.3
Adjust PRF (velocity scale) and baseline in order to avoid aliasing. See Fig. 9.4

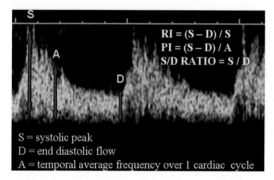

S = systolic peak
D = end diastolic flow
A = temporal average frequency over 1 cardiac cycle

Fig. 9.5 Typical internal carotid artery spectrum. The indices more frequently utilized to describe the flow waveform are explained in the figure

They are described in Fig. 9.5.

Generally speaking, a low-pulsatility waveform is indicative of low distal resistance (e.g., internal carotid), while high-pulsatility waveforms occur in high-resistance vascular beds like the external carotid. The presence of a proximal stenosis, a vascular steal, or an arteriovenous fistula can modify the waveform shape. Care should be taken when trying to interpret indices as absolute measurements of either upstream or downstream flow characteristics. For example, alterations in heart rate can consequently alter the flow waveform shape, determining significant changes in the value of indices.

Practical guidelines to perform a correct spectral analysis are summarized in Table 9.2.

9.1.6 Power Doppler

This technique enables to detect the presence of flow in a selected area independently from the angle and direction of flow (Fig. 9.6) [5]. The amplitude of the signal is dependent only from the density in red blood cells. As compared to color flow imaging, this technique allows a better definition of the marginal signal, and it is not affected by aliasing phenomena. However, it misses information about the direction and velocity of the flow. Therefore, this technique is recommended to evaluate slow flow vessels and to study small or deeper vessels, hardly described by color Doppler.

9.2 Clinical Application

9.2.1 Neuroradiology

Echo color Doppler of extracranial vessels is the examination of choice for the diagnosis and follow-up of cerebrovascular diseases [1, 3]. In asymptomatic patients, ECD examination is helpful to identify subjects at risk of stroke, particularly in those patients who suffer from multiple cardiovascular risk factors.

In patients with neurological signs of cerebral ischemia, instead, echo color Doppler is helpful to identify and control carotid anomalies, such as plaques, that can cause hemodynamic stenosis or

Fig. 9.6 Color imaging with color flow (**a**) and power Doppler (**b**) of internal carotid. Note in **a** the *blue color* in the carotid bulb (*green arrow*) suggestive of nonlaminar flow. In **b**, power Doppler shows only different shades of *red*, indicative of density of red blood cell (the *red arrow* shows the color scale). Because this technique lacks indication about flow direction, the color remains red (*green arrow*)

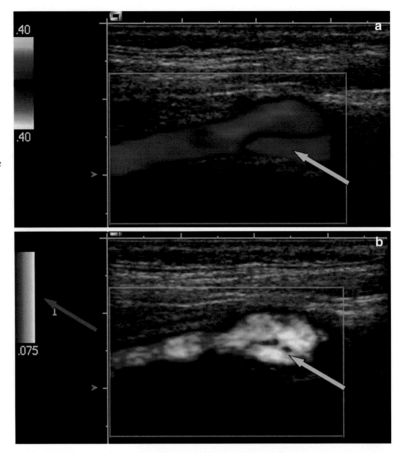

occlusions, dissections, or thromboembolism. Additionally, ECD has an important role in identifying flow reversal conditions, such as in the case of subclavian steal syndrome, steno-occlusive disease of the proximal subclavian artery with retrograde flow in the ipsilateral vertebral artery, and associated cerebral ischemic symptoms. The main neurological application of ECD is summarized in Table 9.3.

9.2.2 Neurosurgery

Intraoperative transdural Doppler ultrasonography (ioTDUS) enables to directly evaluate brain tumors or vascular lesions during operations [6–12]. The advantage is to obtain a real-time visualization of the tumor vascularization, the feeding arteries, and the draining veins of the lesion, while at the same time evaluating the dis-

placement of the normal angioarchitecture; thus, ioTDUS helps obtain safer resection of the lesions, and preserve the normal vessels. It can be routinely performed before opening the dura, after the morphological B-mode imaging. The three main ECD techniques, i.e. color flow, spectral Doppler, and power Doppler, are usefully utilized to correctly assess the tumor vascularization and its relationship with the adjacent brain vessels.

Color Doppler in the B-mode image, identifying the presence and the direction of the flow, can be successfully applied in case of surgical disconnection of an arteriovenous fistula or in bypass surgery.

Power Doppler can present some advantage when applied in meningioma and glioma surgery (Fig. 9.7), due to its capability to correctly visualize deep low-flow vessels, feeding arteries, and neighboring vital vessels.

Table 9.3 ECD study: main neurological indications

		Echo B-mode	Color flow	Spectral Doppler
Atheromatous pathology	Carotid thickening	Identification and measurement of vessel thickenings.	Normal	Normal
	Not significant plaques	Morphology (ulcerations, irregularities) and echogenicity (lipidic/fibrous/calcific) of atheromasic plaques. Visualization of patent (anhechoic) lumen (less useful in case of calcific plaques with shadow)	Color filling of the residual lumen	Normal
	Hemodynamic plaques	Possible visualization of residual lumen	Aliasing phenomena. Upstream and downstream turbolence phenomena	Flow acceleration. Possible aliasing phenomena. Upstream and downstream flow modifications
	Vessel Occlusion	Possible direct visualization of the occluding thrombus	Absent flow downstream the occlusion	Absent flow downstream the occlusion. Upstream high resistance flow
Cervical vessels dissections		Possible visualization of intimal flap, proximal ICA hematoma or low reflective thrombus	Possible visualization of two differently colored compartments along the vessel representing real and false lumen	upstream high resistance flow
Aneurysms of cervical arteries		Circular anechoic formation along the course of the vessel	Circular image detected in transversal sections separated in 2 differently colored areas (the darkest colors can be found in the aneurysmal sac representing slow flow)	No utility
Radiant Therapy/arterities affecting cervical arteries		Hypoechoic vessel thickenings. Vessels narrowing with possible focal stenosis	Varies according to the presence of focal stenosis	Varies according to the presence of focal stenosis

Findings according to the different techniques utilized

Fig. 9.7 IoTDUS power Doppler to evaluate surrounding vascular structures in a case of an fronto-opercular high-grade glioma, showing the draining veins towards the periventricular zone (*white arrows*)

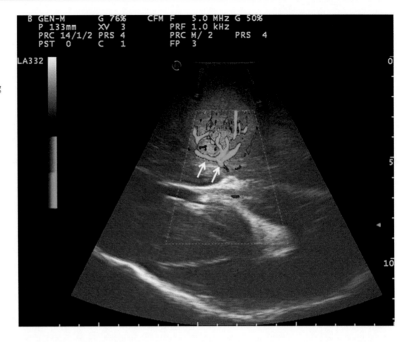

Fig. 9.8 IoTDUS – color flow and spectral Doppler applied to evaluate the superior sagittal sinus (SSS) in a case of a large parasagittal meningioma, showing venous flow around the SSS (*arrow*)

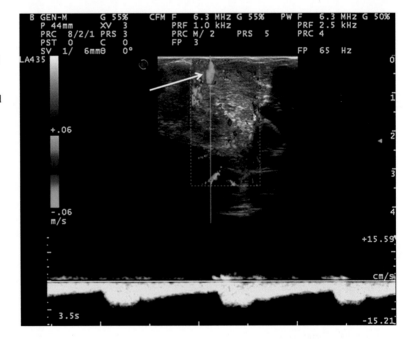

Spectral Doppler is usually combined with B-mode and Doppler technique to asses flow parameters of the surrounding vessels by monitoring the persistence of normal flow during the surgical resection of the lesion (Figs. 9.8 and 9.9). The main limitations are still the angle dependency and the lack of anatomical information; as in color Doppler, adjustments in *PRF*, *IA*, and *gain* must be set before and during the study registration.

Fig. 9.9 IoTDUS – color flow and spectral Doppler to evaluate surrounding vascular structures in a case of a fronto-opercular high-grade glioma. Pulsate Doppler analysis is focused on a terminal branch of the middle cerebral artery (*white arrow*) exiting the Sylvian fissure. Note the typical spectrum of a low resistance vessel flow, characteristic of the vessels of the circle of Willis (*blue arrow*)

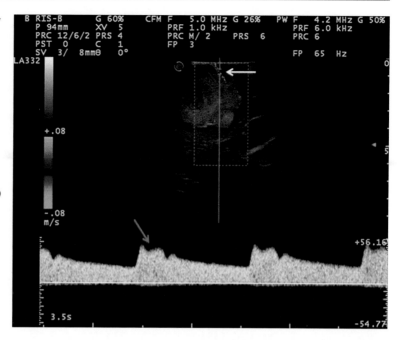

In conclusion, important information that can be obtained with ioTDUS during surgery are as follows:

1. The presence or absence of a Doppler signal (with power or color Doppler) that demonstrates whether the vessel is patent or not.
2. Flow direction detected by color flow.
3. The absolute flow velocity that can be estimated according to the spectral Doppler.
4. Presence of vessel stenosis, with local flow acceleration or, in preocclusive cases, with total flow velocity reduction.
5. The peripheral resistance in normal and in pathological cases, such as in artificial hypotension, hyperemia, and arteriosclerosis. Abnormal peripheral resistance is characterized by the alteration of the ratio between the systolic and diastolic amplitude.
6. Flow irregularities and turbulences due to acceleration and wall irregularities that produce typical Doppler flow patterns, with broadening of the spectrum and irregular curves of the maximum and mean velocities.

Finally, fusion image technique between ioTDUS and volumetric MRI (Fig. 9.10) allows to obtain a more precise vascular map of the surgical area, increasing the neuronavigation accuracy and making the surgical resection safer.

9.2.3 Transcranial Doppler Ultrasound

Transcranial Doppler (TCD), first described in 1982 [13], is a noninvasive ultrasound technique that implies the use of a low-frequency (≤ 2 MHz) probe to study major basal cerebral arteries through bone windows [14]. TCD allows to perform a prolonged continuous monitoring of cerebral blood flow velocities, thus providing complementary information in terms of hemodynamic patterns when used in combination with other neuroradiological techniques (i.e., CT angiography, MR angiography, digital subtraction angiography (DSA)) [15]. The main limitations are the operator dependency and the potentially inadequate transtemporal acoustic window (10–20 % of subjects) [14, 16, 17]. On the other hand, the introduction of technologies such as transcranial color-coded duplex (TCCD) and power motion mode (PMD, M-mode) has further simplified the correct detection of

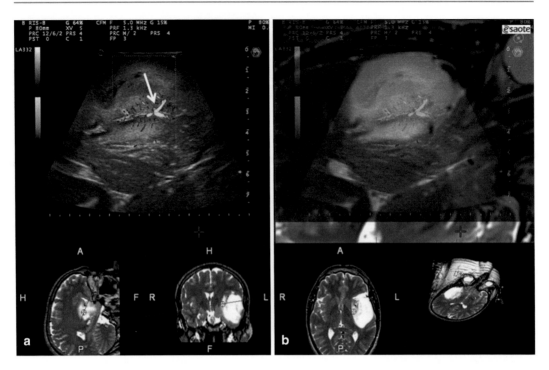

Fig. 9.10 Intraoperative tumor visualization with trans-dural power Doppler with fusion imaging between real-time ultrasound (**a**) and preoperative T2-weighted MRI . The technique is useful to evaluate the vascularization pattern in a case of a large left temporo-insular low-grade glioma. The arterial supply to the internal portion of the tumor is supplied from the middle cerebral artery by many perforating branches (*white arrow*)

cerebral blood flow velocity [18, 19]. Furthermore, the occurrence of altered cardiac outflow, as well as the presence of structural irregularities of the intracranial distal and/or extracranial proximal arteries may characterize an overestimation or underestimation of the intracranial blood flow values. Normally, four acoustic windows exist: transtemporal, suboc-cipital, transorbital, and submandibular (retro-mandibular). Middle (MCA, M1-M2 segments), anterior (ACA, A1 segment), posterior cerebral (PCA, P1–P2 segments), and terminal internal carotid arteries are insonated through the trans-temporal window. Ophthalmic artery and inter-nal carotid siphon are insonated through the transorbital window. Vertebral (VA, intracranial segment) and basilar arteries (BA) are insonated through the suboccipital window. Distal (extra-cranial) internal carotid artery (ICA) is insonated through the submandibular window.

9.2.3.1 Main TCD Parameters

Mean flow velocity (MFV) is a key factor in TCD. Modifications of MFV in the basal cerebral arteries may depend on several physiological parameters (i.e., age, sex, pregnancy, mean arte-rial pressure, hematocrit, PCO_2) [20, 21], and they should always be correlated with the under-lying clinical condition which TCD had been performed for. Standard depth of insonation, flow direction, and normal MFV were described else-where [22]. Pulsatility index (PI) and resistivity index (RI) give information on downstream cere-bral vascular resistance. PI is usually normal between 0.5 and 1.19 [23], whereas RI >0.8 indi-cates increased downstream resistance. The MCA (MFV)/extracranial ICA (MFV) is known as the Lindegaard ratio (LR). It is important in the conditions related to increase of flow veloci-ties (i.e., hyperdynamic flow [<3] and vasospasm [>3]) [24, 25]. A modified LR (BA [MFV]/aver-

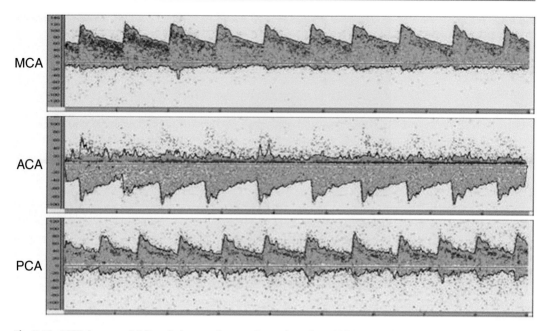

Fig. 9.11 TCD (transcranial Doppler): normal spectral waveform from MCA (M1 segment – middle cerebral artery), ACA (A1 segment – anterior cerebral artery) and PCA (P1 segment – posterior cerebral artery)

age of left and right extracranial VA [MFV]) >3 indicates severe BA vasospasm [25, 26].

9.2.3.2 Transcranial Doppler Equipment

TCD (Fig. 9.11): it can be considered as a non-duplex transcranial Doppler. Standard criteria exist to assess blood flow velocities from specific arteries. Since Doppler signal is "blind," the window used, orientation of the probe, direction of the blood flow, and depth of insonation must be necessarily known. Furthermore, a response to definite maneuvers (as common carotid artery compression) may help in the correct evaluation and recognition of the intracranial artery. More recently, the power M-mode TCD provided multi-gate flow information, thus displaying flow signals at the same time. It might facilitate the temporal window location and the blood flow velocity assessment of multiple vessels.

TCCD (Fig. 9.12): it can be considered as a duplex equipment. Identification of the arteries is allowed by the combination of view of the area of insonation with the pulsed wave Doppler. Basing on different anatomic locations, TCCD can there-fore quite simply help the detection of intracranial arteries. Furthermore, as compared to TCD, flow velocities may be more properly evaluated because the angle of insonation can be measured.

9.3 Main Clinical Applications

9.3.1 Vasospasm after Subarachnoid Hemorrhage (SAH)

After aneurysmal SAH, angiographic cerebral vasospasm (VSP) often occurs. Two-thirds of subjects with SAH have VSP and 50 % of them become symptomatic. VSP severity after SAH is strictly correlated with flow velocities in most cerebral arteries, even though this link appears to be less strong for ACA and ICA [27].

Proximal VSP in any intracranial artery is more easily detectable than distal VSP, with TCD. Increase of flow velocities due to proximal VSP in the intracranial arteries is not followed by a comparable flow velocity increase in the extra-cranial arteries (carotid or the vertebral arteries).

Fig. 9.12 TCCD
(transcranial color-coded
duplex): insonation of MCA
(middle cerebral artery)

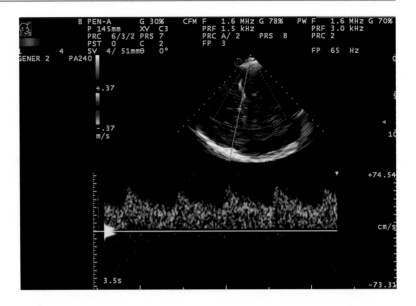

Delayed VSP has great implications on morbidity and mortality. About 25 % of subjects with SAH develop ischemic deficit due to VSP [16, 20, 28, 29].

DSA is the gold standard for VSP diagnosis, but TCD can noninvasively monitor the vasospasm during the therapy and evaluate its efficacy.

TCD has a high sensitivity and specificity in case of MCA and BA VSP [27]. An accurate prediction of absence or presence of angiographic MCA VSP may be identified with MFV patterns <120 cm/s and >200 cm/s, respectively. LR between 3 and 6 is a sign of mild VSP and >6 is an indication of severe VSP [30].

For the detection of >50 % BA VSP, TCD has a sensitivity of 92 % and specificity of 97 % [26], when MFV >85 cm/s and modified LR >3. In case of MFV >95 cm/s, specificity could go up to 100 % [31].

Although evidence of prognostic implication is limited, TCD is a reasonable tool to monitor the development of vasospasm after SAH [32].

9.3.2 Traumatic Brain Injury and Raised Intracranial Pressure (ICP)

Traumatic brain injury (TBI) is one of the leading causes of death and disability. Cerebral vascular injury and hemodynamic compromise, due to raised intracranial pressure, may considerably contribute to poor outcome in subjects with TBI.

TBI complications may lead to four different phases: hypoperfusion (day 0), hyperemia (days 1–3), vasospasm (days 4–15), and raised ICP [32]. TCD may provide prognostic information after TBI by the identification of hemodynamic changes after head injury [20, 27].

Early TCD monitoring can help the physician to prevent cerebral hypoperfusion, thus trying to avoid the extent of secondary ischemic injuries in TBI subjects with raised ICP.

9.3.3 Cerebral Circulatory Arrest and Brain Death

A decrease in cerebral perfusion pressure and a simultaneous increase in intracranial pressure support the cessation of brain flow by compression of the intracranial arteries. The lack of brain flow may therefore lead to cerebral circulatory arrest (CCA) [16].

TCD may continuously monitor the cerebral blood flow, thus supporting the diagnosis of CCA and brain death. Classical TCD spectral waveform abnormalities related to raised ICP and CCA are an oscillating "to-and-fro" movement of blood flow (attributed to reversal of flow in diastole), as well as small early systolic spikes [33, 34].

Since TCD has a very high sensitivity (96.5 %) and specificity (100 %) in the diagnosis of CCA [35], it is considered a useful confirmatory test of brain death together with clinical, neuroradiological, and neurophysiological tests [36]. Furthermore, when EEG is unreliable due to pharmacological sedation, TCD may be more useful for CCA diagnosis [37].

9.3.4   Sickle Cell Disease

Chronic hemolysis in children with sickle cell disease (SCD) provokes a low hemoglobin content, thus leading to hypoxia by chronic anemia, with consequent angiogenesis and neovascularization. This vascular system characterized by chronic inflammation due to the adherence of sickled cells to the pathological endothelium results in ischemic and hemorrhagic infarcts [38]. Intracranial arterial stenosis and/or occlusion are mostly present at distal ICA, proximal MCA, and ACA.

TCD screening of children (2–6 years old) is recommended. An increased risk of stroke of 10,000 per 100,000 patient-years in asymptomatic children with SCD is present when MCA or ICA MFV >200 cm/s [39, 40].

Nowadays, TCD monitoring and regular transfusion in those children with SCD and high TCD flow velocities are considered a standard of care [27].

9.3.5   Microemboli Detection-Carotid Stenosis

TCD is the only medical device able to detect cerebral microemboli, both solid and gaseous, in real time. Embolic signals by TCD are usually found in specific conditions related to cardioembolic diseases and aortic and extracranial and intracranial atheromatosis, during diagnostic procedures (i.e., DSA, coronary artery catheterization) as well as during therapeutic procedures regarding heart and carotid diseases. Among all several conditions in which TCD is involved as technique for emboli detection, carotid stenosis is one of the most com-

monly considered. Furthermore, apart from emboli detection, TCD may allow a real-time monitoring of flow velocities.

TCD may identify asymptomatic embolic signals in subjects with carotid artery disease. Moreover, those patients with asymptomatic carotid stenosis may be considered at high or low risk of future stroke, basing on the presence or lack of embolization, respectively [41]. Furthermore, TCD identification of asymptomatic embolization in subjects with both symptomatic and asymptomatic carotid artery stenosis can be considered an independent predictor of ischemic stroke [42]. TCD monitoring during carotid endarterectomy and carotid stenting provides information about embolization and flow patterns in order to reduce the intraoperative risk of stroke.

9.3.6   Microemboli Detection-Patent Foramen Ovale (PFO)

About 30 % of adults have a patent foramen ovale (PFO), but the frequency is higher (approximately 50 %) in patients with cerebral infarct of unknown etiology, especially in the young people [43–46]. Even if transesophageal echocardiography is considered the gold standard for PFO diagnosis, contrast-enhanced TCD provides high sensitivity in the right-to-left shunt (RLS) diagnosis due to PFO [47]. TCD has the advantage to be noninvasive, does not require sedation for the Valsalva maneuver, provides direct evidence of emboli passage through the cerebral arteries, and may be performed both in adults and children without noteworthy difficulties. The more RLS, the higher is the patency of the foramen ovale (Fig. 9.13). It is important to point out that not every RLS is related to PFO (i.e., pulmonary arteriovenous fistula). In the latter condition, TCD may not clearly discriminate between PFO and pulmonary arteriovenous fistula.

PFO is a contraindication for semi-sitting/sitting position in neurosurgical procedures [48]. TCD may allow RLS detection in those subjects who undergo these procedures. TCD results might help the anesthetist in a prompt management during all phases of the neurosurgical intervention.

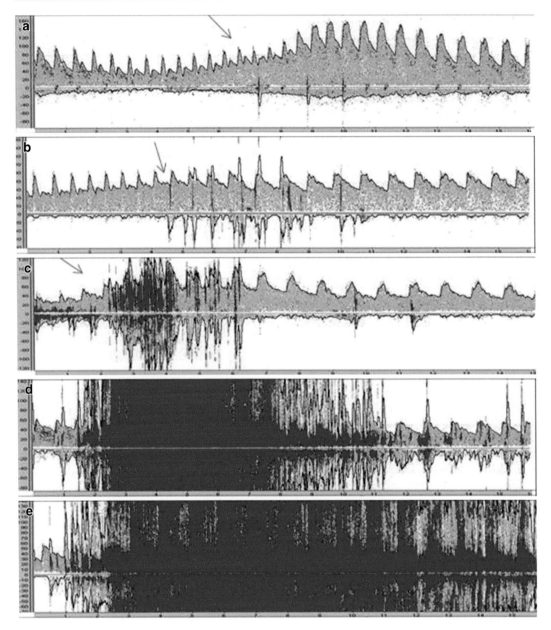

Fig. 9.13 TCD (transcranial Doppler). Evaluation of right-to-left shunt (RLS). Five different RLS patterns (a–e). (a–c) single-spikes pattern with (a) a noticeable Valsalva maneuver (see *arrow*), (b, c) single spikes (see *arrows*); (d, e) shower-curtain pattern indicating a huge RLS (uncountable spikes)

9.3.7 Ischemic Stroke

TCD is useful in acute ischemic stroke, determining the vascular patency of intracranial arteries. Repeated TCD studies may track the course of an arterial occlusion before and after treatment (i.e., thrombolysis). Initiation, speed, timing, and degree of recanalization can consistently be detected by TCD flow changes [49]. Detection of acute MCA occlusions by TCD has high (>90 %) sensitivity, specificity, and positive (PPV) and negative predictive values (NPV) [50–53]. Acute occlusion in the ICA siphon and vertebral and basilar arteries by TCD presents lesser sensitivity (70–90 %) and PPV and high specificity and NPV (>90 %) [54].

Parameters of evaluation for acute ischemic stroke and arterial occlusion, as TIBI (thrombolysis in brain ischemia) [55] and COGIF (consensus on grading intracranial flow obstruction) [56], correlate well with the initial stroke severity, mortality, likelihood of reperfusion, and clinical improvement. Furthermore, plenty of microembolic signals on TCD can suggest the earlier start of a specific treatment (i.e., anticoagulation or antiplatelet agents), and hyperemic flow pattern can help the physician to modify blood pressure [57]. In addition, early TCD findings can be very useful for prognosis in patients with acute ischemic stroke. In these patients, intracranial arterial occlusion detected by TCD is associated with poor 90-day outcome [58, 59], whereas a normal TCD study is predictive of early recovery [60, 61]. Since ultrasound exposure enhances both spontaneous and thrombolytic agent-mediated lysis of intravascular clot, TCD monitoring was used to improve the arterial recanalization after an ischemic stroke within 2 h following tPA bolus [62]. Enhancement of tPA-associated clot lysis by ultrasound can significantly be augmented by the use of diagnostic microbubbles or lipid microspheres.

TCD is otherwise used for the evaluation of intracranial stenosis.

Intracranial atherosclerosis is a significant risk factor for ischemic strokes and transient ischemic attacks (TIAs) (~10 % of these events) [63, 64]. TCD can be used to detect stenosis, mostly in the anterior circulation [16, 30, 65]. The tortuosity and anatomic variability of the vessels in the posterior circulation reduce TCD sensitivity, specificity, NPV and PPV in the detection of stenosis. MFV cutoffs are 100 and 80 cm/s for >50 % stenosis [66] for MCA and VA/BA, respectively. MFV higher than 120 and 110 cm/s is accepted as an indicator of 70 % stenosis [67] for MCA and VA/BA, respectively. Based on considerable NPV and low PPV for MCA and BA stenosis, TCD may be considered as a reliable technique to rule out an intracranial stenosis [68].

However, TCD abnormal findings in terms of increased flow velocities due to possible intracranial stenosis do not necessarily correlate with clinical implications; a neuroradiological confirmatory test is therefore indicated.

9.3.8 Cerebral Autoregulation

Cerebral autoregulation maintains cerebral blood flow constant between mean arterial pressures of 50 and 170 mmHg. TCD provides continuous measurements of cerebral blood flow velocity in the major basal cerebral arteries and is the most commonly utilized technique to evaluate cerebral blood flow regulation. Abnormalities in cerebral autoregulation occur in several clinical disorders such as stroke, subarachnoid hemorrhage, eclampsia, postpartum angiopathy, syncope, and traumatic brain injury.

9.3.8.1 Cerebral Vasoreactivity (CVR)
The vasodilatory response of the cerebral resistance vessels is known as cerebrovascular reactivity (CVR) and is crucial in cerebrovascular diseases [69, 70]. Increased CO_2 causes arteriolar vasodilatation resulting in increased velocity in the upstream larger cerebral arteries (insonated vessels). Clinical conditions, as intracranial-extracranial stenosis/occlusion may alter CVR, up to an exhausted arteriolar vasodilatation which can put the subject at risk for future ischemic stroke. TCD provides solid information regarding CVR either by breath-holding, CO_2 inhalation, or acetazolamide [71–73].

References

1. Evans DH, Jensen JA, Nielsen MB (2011) Ultrasonic colour Doppler imaging. Interface Focus 1(4):490–502. doi:10.1098/rsfs.2011.0017
2. Wells PN (1994) Ultrasonic colour flow imaging. Phys Med Biol 39(12):2113–2145
3. Evans DH, McDicken WN, Skidmore R, Woodcock JP (1989) Doppler ultrasound: physics, instrumentation, and clinical applications. Wiley, Chichester
4. Kremkau FW (1992) Doppler color imaging. Principles and instrumentation. Clin Diagn Ultrasound 27:7–60, Review

5. Rubin JM (1999) Power Doppler. Eur Radiol 9(Suppl 3):S318–S322

6. Prada F, Del Bene M, Moiraghi A, Casali C, Legnani FG, Saladino A, Perin A, Vetrano IG, Mattei L, Richetta C, Saini M, DiMeco F (2015) From grey scale B-mode to elastosonography: multimodal ultrasound imaging in meningioma surgery—pictorial essay and literature review. BioMed Res Int 2015:925729

7. van Leyen K, Klötzsch C, Harrer JU (2011) Brain tumor imaging with transcranial sonography: state of the art and review of the literature. Ultraschall Med 32(6):572–581. doi:10.1055/s-0031-1273443, Epub 2011 Oct 27

8. Becker G, Perez J, Krone A et al (1992) Transcranial color-coded real-time sonography in the evaluation of intracranial neoplasms and arteriovenous malformations. Neurosurgery 31:420–428

9. Sosna J, Barth MM, Kruskal JB et al (2005) Intraoperative sonography for neurosurgery. J Ultrasound Med 24:1671–1682

10. Unsgaard G, Gronningsaeter A, Ommedal S et al (2002) Brain operations guided by real-time two-dimensional ultrasound: new possibilities as a result of improved image quality. Neurosurgery 51:402–412

11. Becker G, Krone A, Koulis D et al (1994) Reliability of transcranial colour-coded real-time sonography in assessment of brain tumours: correlation of ultrasound, computed tomography and biopsy findings. Neuroradiology 36:585–590

12. Solheim O, Selbekk T, Lindseth F, Unsgard G (2009) Navigated resection of giant intracranial meningiomas based on intraoperative 3D ultrasound. Acta Neurochir (Wien) 151(9):1143–1151. doi:10.1007/s00701-009-0395-1

13. Aaslid R, Markwalder TM, Nornes H (1982) Noninvasive transcranial Doppler ultrasound recording of flow velocity in basal cerebral arteries. J Neurosurg 57(6):769–774

14. Moppett IK, Mahajan RP (2004) Transcranial Doppler ultrasonography in anaesthesia and intensive care. Br J Anaesth 93(5):710–724

15. Topcuoglu MA, Unal A, Arsava EM (2010) Advances in transcranial Doppler clinical applications. Expert Opin Med Diagn 4:343–358

16. Tsivgoulis G, Alexandrov AV, Sloan MA (2009) Advances in transcranial Doppler ultrasonography. Curr Neurol Neurosci Rep 9(1):46–54

17. Marinoni M, Ginanneschi A, Forleo P, Amaducci L (1997) Technical limits in Transcranial Doppler recording: inadequate acoustic windows. Ultrasound Med Biol 23(8):1275–1277

18. Bogdahn U, Becker G, Winkler J, Greiner K, Perez J, Meurers B (1990) Transcranial color-coded real-time sonography in adults. Stroke 21:1680–1688

19. Moehring MA, Spencer MP (2002) Power M-mode Doppler (PMD) for observing cerebral blood flow and tracking emboli. Ultrasound Med Biol 28:49–57

20. White H, Venkatesh B (2006) Applications of transcranial Doppler in the ICU: a review. Intensive Care Med 32(7):981–994

21. Schatlo B, Pluta RM (2007) Clinical applications of transcranial Doppler sonography. Rev Recent Clin Trials 2(1):49–57

22. Alexandrov A, Sloan MA, Wong LK, Douville C, Razumovsky AY, Koroshetz WJ, Kaps M, Tegeler CH (2007) Practice standards for transcranial doppler ultrasound: part I- test Performance. J Neuroimaging 17(1):11–8

23. Gosling RG, King DH (1974) Arterial assessment by Doppler shift ultrasound. Proc Royal Soc Med 67(6, part 1):447–449

24. Lindegaard KF, Nornes H, Bakke SJ, Sorteberg W, Nakstad P (1988) Cerebral vasospasm after subarachnoid haemorrhage investigated by means of Transcranial Doppler ultrasound. Acta Neurochir 42:81–84

25. Aaslid R, Huber P, Nornes H (1984) Evaluation of cerebrovascular spasm with transcranial Doppler ultrasound. J Neurosurg 60(1):37–41

26. Sviri GE, Ghodke B, Britz GW et al (2006) Transcranial Doppler grading criteria for basilar artery vasospasm. Neurosurgery 59(2):360–366

27. Sloan MA, Alexandrov AV, Tegeler CH et al (2004) Therapeutics and Technology Assessment Subcommittee of the American Academy of Neurology. Assessment: transcranial Doppler ultrasonography: report of the Therapeutics and Technology Assessment Subcommittee of the American Academy of Neurology. Neurology 62(9):1468–1481

28. Papaioannou V, Dragoumanis C, Theodorou V, Konstantonis D, Pneumatikos I, Birbilis T (2008) Transcranial Doppler ultrasonography in intensive care unit. Report of a case with subarachnoid hemorrhage and brain death and review of the literature. Greek E J Perioperat Med 6:95–104

29. Biller J, Godersky JC, Adams HP Jr (1988) Management of aneurysmal subarachnoid hemorrhage. Stroke 19(10):1300–1305

30. Lindegaard KF, Nornes H, Bakke SJ, Sorteberg W, Nakstad P (1989) Cerebral vasospasm diagnosis by means of angiography and blood velocity measurements. Acta Neurochir (Wien) 100(1–2):12–24

31. Sloan MA, Burch CM, Wozniak MA et al (1994) Transcranial Doppler detection of vertebrobasilar vasospasm following subarachnoid hemorrhage. Stroke 25(11):2187–2197

32. Connolly JS, Rabinstein AA, Carhuapoma JR (2012) Guidelines for the management of aneurysmal subarachnoid hemorrhage: a guideline for healthcare professionals from the American Heart Association/American Stroke Association. Stroke 43(6):1711–37

33. Feri M, Ralli L, Felici M et al (1994) Transcranial Doppler and brain death diagnosis. Crit Care Med 22(7):1120–1126

34. Yoneda S, Nishimoto A, Nukada T et al (1974) To-and-fro movement and external escape of carotid

arterial blood in brain death cases. A Doppler Ultrasonic Study. Stroke 5(6):707–713

35. Rasulo FA, De Peri E, Lavinio A (2008) Transcranial Doppler ultrasonography in intensive care. Eur J Anaesthesiol Suppl 42(42):167–173

36. Wijdicks EF (1995) Determining brain death in adults. Neurology 45(5):1003–1011

37. Ducrocq X, Hassler W, Moritake K et al (1998) Consensus opinion on diagnosis of cerebral circulatory arrest using Doppler-sonography: task Force Group on cerebral death of the Neurosonology Research Group of the World Federation of Neurology. J Neurol Sci 159(2):145–150

38. Jordan LC, Casella JF, Debaun MR (2012) Prospects for primary stroke prevention in children with sickle cell anaemia. Br J Haematol 9

39. Adams RJ, McKie VC, Carl EM et al (1997) Long-term stroke risk in children with sickle cell disease screened with transcranial Doppler. Ann Neurol 42(5):699–704

40. Adams RJ, Brambilla D (2005) Discontinuing prophylactic transfusions used to prevent stroke in sickle cell disease. N Engl J Med 353:2769–2778

41. Markus HS, King A, Shipley M et al (2010) Asymptomatic embolisation for prediction of stroke in the Asymptomatic Carotid Emboli Study (ACES): a prospective observational study. Lancet Neurol 9(7):663–671

42. Molloy J, Markus HS (1999) Asymptomatic embolization predicts stroke and TIA risk in patients with carotid artery stenosis. Stroke 30(7):1440–1443

43. Hagen PT, Scholz DG, Edwards WD (1984) Incidence and size of patent foramen ovale during the first 10 decades of life: an autopsy study of 965 normal hearts. Mayo Clin Proc 59(1):17–20

44. Adams HP, Bendixen BH, Kappelle LJ et al (1993) Classification of subtype of acute ischemic stroke. Definitions for use in a multicenter clinical trial. TOAST. Trial of Org 10172 in Acute Stroke Treatment. Stroke 24(1):35–41

45. Job FP, Ringelstein EB, Grafen Y et al (1994) Comparison of transcranial contrast Doppler sonography and transesophageal contrast echocardiography for the detection of patent foramen ovale in young stroke patients. Am J Cardiol 74(4):381–384

46. Serena J, Segura T, Perez-Ayuso MJ et al (1998) The need to quantify right-to-left shunt in acute ischemic stroke: a case-control study. Stroke 29(7):1322–1328

47. Caputi L, Carriero MR, Falcone C, Parati E, Piotti P, Materazzo C, Anzola GP (2009) Transcranial Doppler and transesophageal echocardiography: comparison of both techniques and prospective clinical relevance of transcranial Doppler in patent foramen ovale detection. J Stroke Cerebrovasc Dis 18(5):343–348

48. Jadik S, Wissing H, Friedrich K et al (2009) A standardized protocol for the prevention of clinically relevant venous air embolism during neurosurgical interventions in the semisitting position. Neurosurgery 64:533–539

49. Alexandrov AV, Burgin WS, Demchuk AM, El-Mitwalli A, Grotta JC (2001) Speed of intracranial clot lysis with intravenous tissue plasminogen activator therapy: sonographic classification and short-term improvement. Circulation 103:2897–2902

50. Camerlingo M, Casto L, Censori B, Ferraro B, Gazzaniga GC, Mamoli A (1993) Transcranial Doppler in acute ischemic stroke of the middle cerebral artery territories. Acta Neurol Scand 88(2):108–111

51. Zanette EM, Fieschi C, Bozzao L et al (1989) Comparison of cerebral angiography and transcranial Doppler sonography in acute stroke. Stroke 20(7):899–903

52. Baumgartner RW, Mattle HP, Schroth G (1999) Assessment of >/= 50 % and < 50 % intracranial stenoses by transcranial color-coded duplex sonography. Stroke 30(1):87–92

53. Fieschi C, Argentino C, Lenzi GL, Sacchetti ML, Toni D, Bozzao L (1989) Clinical and instrumental evaluation of patients with ischemic stroke within the first six hours. J Neurol Sci 91(3):311–321

54. Demchuk AM, Christou I, Wein TH et al (2000) Accuracy and criteria for localizing arterial occlusion with transcranial Doppler. J Neuroimaging 10(1):1–12

55. Demchuk AM, Burgin WS, Christou I, Felberg RA, Barber PA, Hill MD, Alexandrov AV (2001) Thrombolysis in brain ischemia (TIBI) transcranial Doppler flow grades predict clinical severity, early recovery, and mortality in patients treated with intravenous tissue plasminogen activator. Stroke 32:89–93

56. Nedelmann M, Stolz E, Gerriets T, Baumgartner RW, Malferrari G, Seidel G, Kaps M (2009) Consensus recommendations for transcranial color-coded duplex sonography for the assessment of intracranial arteries in clinical trials on acute stroke. Stroke 40:3238–3244

57. Burgin WS, Malkoff M, Felberg RA, Demchuk AM, Christou I, Grotta JC, Alexandrov AV (2000) Transcranial Doppler ultrasound criteria for recanalization after thrombolysis for middle cerebral artery stroke. Stroke 31:1128–1132

58. Camerlingo M, Casto L, Censori B, Servalli MC, Ferraro B, Mamoli A (1996) Prognostic use of ultrasonography in acute non-hemorrhagic carotid stroke. Ital J Neurol Sci 17(3):215–218

59. Baracchini C, Manara R, Ermani M, Meneghetti G (2000) The quest for early predictors of stroke evolution: can TCD be a guiding light? Stroke 31(12):2942–2947

60. Kushner MJ, Zanette EM, Bastianello S et al (1991) Transcranial Doppler in acute hemispheric brain infarction. Neurology 41(1):109–113

61. Toni D, Fiorelli M, Zanette EM et al (1998) Early spontaneous improvement and deterioration of ischemic stroke patients. A serial study with transcranial Doppler ultrasonography. Stroke 29(6):1144–1148

62. Alexandrov AV, Molina CA, Grotta JC et al (2004) Ultrasound enhanced systemic thrombolysis for acute ischemic stroke. N Engl J Med 351:2170–2178

63. Sacco RL, Kargman DE, Gu Q, Zamanillo MC (1995) The Northern Manhattan Stroke Study. Race ethnicity and determinants of intracranial atherosclerotic cerebral infarction. Stroke 26(1):14–20

64. Wityk RJ, Lehman D, Klag M, Coresh J, Ahn H, Litt B (1996) Race and sex differences in the distribution of cerebral atherosclerosis. Stroke 27(11):1974–1980

65. Babikian VL, Feldmann E, Wechsler LR et al (2000) Transcranial Doppler ultrasonography: year 2000 update. J Neuroimaging 10(2):101–115

66. Feldmann E, Wilterdink JL, Kosinski A et al (2007) The stroke outcomes and neuroimaging of intracranial atherosclerosis (SONIA) trial. Neurology 68:2099–2106

67. Chimowitz MI, Lynn MJ, Derdeyn CP et al (2011) Stenting versus aggressive medical therapy for intracranial arterial stenosis. N Engl J Med 365:993–1003

68. Zhao L, Barlinn K, Sharma VK et al (2011) Velocity criteria for intracranial stenosis revisited n international multicenter study of transcranial Doppler and digital subtraction angiography. Stroke 42:3429–3434

69. Markus H, Cullinane M (2001) Severely impaired cerebrovascular reactivity predicts stroke and TIA risk in patients with carotid artery stenosis and occlusion. Brain 124(3):457–467

70. Vernieri F, Pasqualetti P, Passarelli F, Rossini PM, Silvestrini M (1999) Outcome of carotid artery occlusion is predicted by cerebrovascular reactivity. Stroke 30(3):593–598

71. Marshall RS, Rundek T, Sproule DM et al (2003) Monitoring of cerebral vasodilatory capacity with transcranial Doppler carbon dioxide inhalation in patients with severe carotid artery disease. Stroke 34(4):945–949

72. Ogasawara K, Ogawa A, Yoshimoto T (2002) Cerebrovascular reactivity to acetazo-lamide and outcome in patients with symptomatic internal carotid or middle cerebral artery occlusion: a xenon-133 single-photon emission computed tomography study. Stroke 33(7):1857–1862

73. Markus HS, Harrison MJ (1992) Estimation of cerebrovascular reactivity using trans-cranial Doppler, including the use of breath-holding as the vasodilatory stimulus. Stroke 23(5):668–673

Part IV

Intra-operative Ultrasound, Fusion Imaging and Virtual Navigation

Virtual Navigation and Interventional Procedures

10

Giovanni Mauri and Luigi Solbiati

10.1 Introduction

Image-guided interventional procedures are playing an increasingly important role for a diverse set of therapies, from endovascular procedures to percutaneous thermal ablation [7, 28, 32, 54], medical fields for which imaging plays a crucial role. The optimal visualization of patient's anatomy, treatment target, and devices used is of paramount importance for achieving the best clinical results. Over the last several years, the technological advancement of imaging modalities has been impressive. Modern computed tomography (CT) scanners allow for a complete cardiac scan in less than one second with reduced radiation dose [10, 21]. Thanks to 3T magnets, it is possible to achieve incredibly defined magnetic resonance (MR) images [5, 43], and high real-time image quality is currently a standard in ultrasound equipment [6, 63]. However, intrinsic limitations still exist for

most if not all imaging modalities. Thus, besides developing further technological advancements for each single modality, a complementary strategy has been proposed, i.e., fusing information obtained from different imaging modalities in order to overcome the limitations of individual modalities [3, 8, 30, 31, 34, 39, 42, 64]. In diagnostic imaging, this concept has led to the birth of hybrid CT and positron emission tomography (PET) scanners, which provide, in a single examination, high-quality anatomic information (thanks to CT) merged with functional information deriving from different tracers detected by PET scanners [1, 8, 36]. In interventional radiology, fusion of real-time ultrasound (US) with CT, MR, or even CT/PET images has been reported as being not only feasible but also effective in guiding percutaneous biopsies and ablations through the body and is thought to be one of the main improvements that will propel the future of interventional radiology [3, 26, 30, 41, 62].

G. Mauri (✉)
Department of Radiology, Policlinico San Donato, San Donato Milanese (Milano), Italy

Department of Interventional Radiology, European Institute of Oncology, Milano, Italy
e-mail: vanni.mauri@gmail.com

L. Solbiati
Department of Biomedical Sciences, Humanitas University, Department of Radiology, Humanitas Research Hospital, Rozzano (Milano), Italy

10.2 Image Guidance for Interventional Biopsies and Ablation

The ideal imaging modality for the guidance of percutaneous biopsies and ablation should provide:

© Springer International Publishing Switzerland 2016
F. Prada et al. (eds.), *Intraoperative Ultrasound (IOUS) in Neurosurgery: From Standard B-mode to Elastosonography*, DOI 10.1007/978-3-319-25268-1_10

- Excellent visualization of the target in all the phases of the procedure
- Excellent visualization and discrimination of the surrounding anatomical structures
- High-definition visualization of the interventional device
- Real-time capabilities to enable detection of device insertion and procedure monitoring
- Ease of use
- Wide availability
- Minimal biologic effects (radiation)
- Low economic cost

Several imaging modalities are currently available for the guidance of percutaneous, diagnostic, and therapeutic interventional procedures, each with various advantages and limitations (Table 10.1).

Sonography (US) is by far the most widely used guidance modality, as it is widely available and relatively inexpensive, allowing for real-time visualization and providing high-spatial resolution. On the other hand, US is a highly operator-dependent technique, has limited field of view, and can be hampered by anatomical structures and obscuring tissue properties such as bones or gas-containing structures. Moreover, for some targets US may have low conspicuity even when ultrasound contrast agents are employed [23, 38, 48, 54–56].

CT is widely used to guide interventional procedures in some countries and is almost mandatory for procedures involving lung or bone. CT provides wider visualization of anatomical structures surrounding the target, and clear visualization of the interventional device, but has also important limitations: the use of ionizing radiation, challenging real-time capability, and difficulty of visualizing an "off-axis" approach. Moreover, conspicuity of the target lesion is often related to the administration of contrast media that, unlike contrast-enhanced US (CEUS), is burdened by dose-related issues [9, 14, 24, 44, 45, 57].

MRI-guided percutaneous interventions can be performed with dedicated scanners (e.g., open or wide-bore systems) and dedicated MRI-compatible devices. Owing to a host of potentially beneficial different sequences and contrast agents for enhancement, targets can be optimally visualized. Yet, the difficult procedural environment and the elevated costs of dedicated MRI systems and compatible devices strongly limit the diffusion of MRI as an image guidance modality [37, 46, 50, 53].

PET and CT/PET have been recently proposed as guidance modalities for percutaneous interventional procedures. Their main advantage is the capability of providing functional information enabling to target the most vital part of a lesion for biopsy or ablation. However, the still limited number of CT/PET scanners, the high costs of the examination, and the elevated radiation dose limit their diffusion as guidance modalities for interventional procedures [49, 51, 58, 60].

As the ideal characteristics are not present in a single imaging modality, usually the expert interventional radiologist "mentally" fuses the information provided by different preacquired imaging modalities while performing the procedure. However, for complex procedures this cerebral process of synthesis can often become quite challenging. Systems that automatically display all the required images simultaneously and in real time, such as modern image fusion equipment and virtual navigation, hold the potential to substantially optimize the efficacy of percutaneous interventional procedures and hold the distinct promise of lessening the dependence from operator experience.

Table 10.1 Characteristics of different imaging modalities for the guidance of percutaneous biopsies and ablations

	US	CT	MR	CT/PET
Target visualization	+	++	++	+++
Surrounding structure visualization	+	+++	+++	+++
Device visualization	++	+++	++	+++
Real-time capability	+++	+	–	–
Ease of use	+++	+	+	+
Availability	+++	++	+	+
Biologic cost	–	+	–	++
Economic cost	+	++	+++	+++

10.3   Fusion Imaging

At the present time several systems are available to perform image fusion and virtual navigation to guide interventional procedures. For all of them the crucial element is the real-time capability, which requires a continuous and fast update of imaging data for real-time co-registration and dynamic image fusion. Systems become more complex when multiple image datasets have to be managed and real-time device tracking is required [1, 3, 40].

The basis and first crucial step of any image fusion system is the correct and precise space alignment of multiple imaging datasets provided by different modalities, the so-called co-registration. To achieve this goal, a virtual three-dimensional (3D) space must be created and overlaid to the real 3D space, in order to achieve the exact correspondence between imaging and real patient [3]. This virtual space is generally created by systems with a hardware and a software integrated in a US machine. The hardware consists in an electromagnetic field generator positioned as close as possible to the area of interest and electromagnetic sensors applicable to different tools (US probes and interventional devices) and recognized by the software in order to detect their relative position in relation to the virtual space achieved (Fig. 10.1a) [4, 26, 30, 47, 62]. Other systems are based on optical recogni-

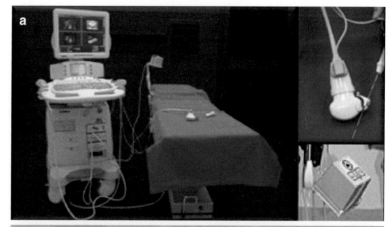

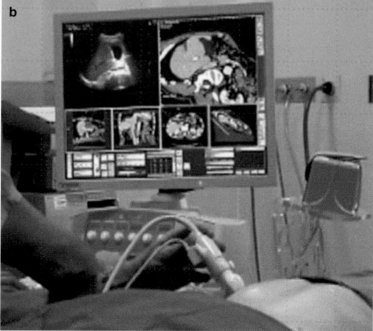

Fig. 10.1 (**a**) Virtual navigation system for real-time US-CT/MR image fusion. The system is made of an US scanner with a dedicated built-in hardware and software (Esaote, Genova, Italy). On the right, the US probe with the electromagnetic sensor applied (*top*) and the magnetic field transmitter (*bottom*). (**b**) After co-registration, US real-time images and the corresponding CT cross-sectional images are simultaneously showed on the US machine screen

Fig. 10.2 System for virtual navigation system based on optical registration (Cascination, Bern, Switzerland). The system is based on an optical camera that is able to recognize some markers applied on the skin of the patient. Once the target has been identified and marked on the reference images, the system provides a path prediction and a system for needle guidance (Courtesy of Dr. A. Michos, Department of Radiology, Danderyd Hospital, Stockholm, Sweden)

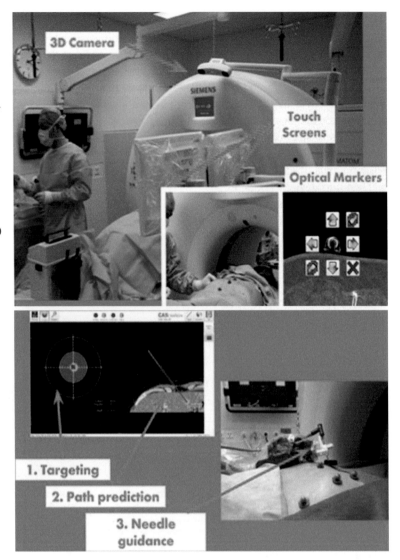

tion of the virtual space and of the different devices to be used during interventional procedures (Figs. 10.2, 10.3, and 10.4) [3, 16, 17, 61].

In order to enable the software to fuse image datasets and achieve a good co-registration, one or more same reference points recognizable in all the datasets used must be identified. These points can be either manually detected (e.g., fiducial markers applied to the skin of patients before acquiring the first image dataset or anatomical landmarks) or, more recently, automatically identified by the system [3, 25]. The employment of external fiducial markers has the limitation of not allowing to use previously acquired imaging data-

sets, for example, in case of patients coming from different hospitals, or when imaging was performed before planning an interventional procedure. When internal markers are employed, previously acquired images can be used. Theoretically, any anatomical structure clearly identifiable in both image datasets to be fused could be used as internal marker, but in order to provide precise co-registration in all the three dimensions, anatomical markers must be as small as possible, like single blood vessels or vessel bifurcations. Automatic registration is based on the automatic recognition by the software of similarities in voxels in two different image datasets.

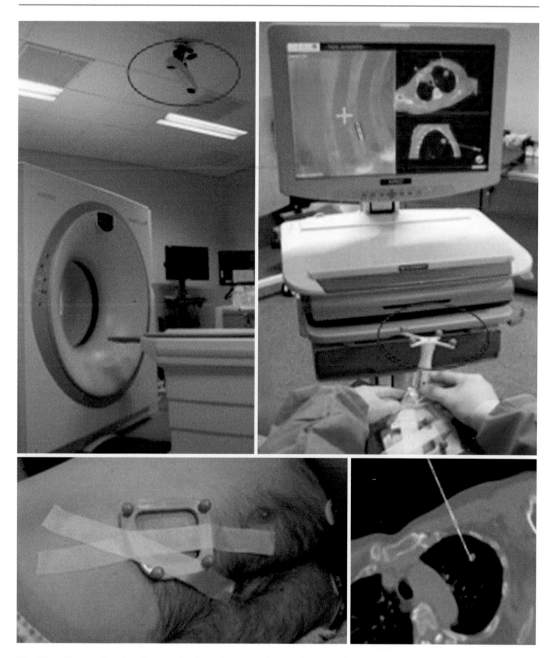

Fig. 10.3 System for virtual navigation based on optical registration for the application in the lung (Sirio, Masmec Biomed, Modugno, Italy). The optical navigation system is based on infrared light reflected by passive spheres available on the needle handle and on the patient's chest (Courtesy of Dr. F. Grasso, Policlinico Universitario Campus Biomedico, Rome, Italy)

In the liver the automatic recognition of blood vessels in three dimensions in the two image datasets to be fused allows for a precise and fast co-registration [3, 25]. Whatever the method used, the co-registered images have subsequently to be displayed in real time during the procedures (Fig. 10.1b). When multiple image datasets (e.g., US, CT, and PET images) have been fused, systems allow to shift rapidly from one dataset to the other or to simultaneously show all the images fused.

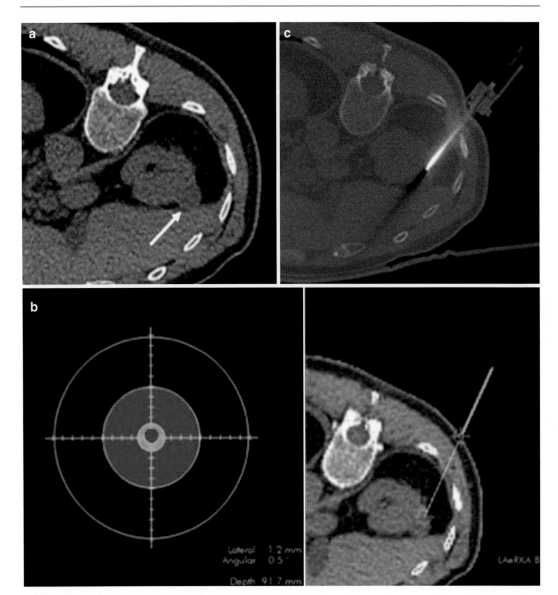

Fig. 10.4 Biopsy of a renal mass with the use of an optical virtual navigation system. (**a**) CT scan of the patient with the target renal lesion (*arrow*). (**b**) Targeting of the lesion under the control of the virtual navigation system. (**c**) CT scan confirming the correct localization of the biopsy device (Courtesy of Dr. A. Michos, Department of Radiology, Danderyd Hospital, Stockholm, Sweden)

10.4 Virtual Navigation

When these steps have been completed, it is possible to "navigate" the virtual space with different tools. A virtual device can be created, corresponding exactly to the real device that is used, whose position can be shown in the 3D virtual space or even overlaid on the real-time imaging of the patient achieved during the procedure.

Whatever system is used, virtual navigation allows for a series of very useful tools. First of all, multiple different markers can be placed at any desired point on a reference image. For example, a target point can be selected on the reference imaging (e.g., CT, MR, or PET) and then showed on the real-time US images (Fig. 10.5b). This allows for the identification of the area where the target is located even when US is not

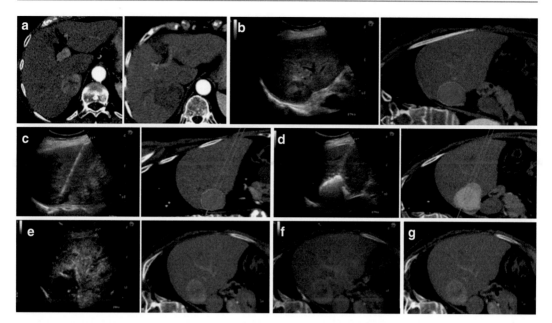

Fig. 10.5 (**a**) CT scan in arterial phase shows a hypervascular rounded mass (hepatocellular carcinoma) at segment VII, in cirrhotic liver. (**b**) With fusion imaging, after co-registration, on CT (*right*) the mass is manually demarcated (*yellow line*) and colored in blue. The corresponding lesion is visualized in the co-registered US scan (*left*). (**c**) Thanks to the application of an electromagnetic sensor to the hub of the microwave antenna used for ablation, during the insertion into the target, the antenna is visible both on US (real device) (*left*) and on CT (virtual device, green parallel lines) (*right*). (**d**) Given the large size of the mass, multiple insertions are required for complete ablation. Following the first insertion, all the subsequent insertions are performed under the guidance of the "virtual needle" because the "cloud" of gas produced by the ablation prevents the visualization of the real device on US (*left image*). Based on preacquired data, the size of the volume of necrosis achievable with each insertion is represented as a green-colored sphere, overlapped by the fusion system over the blue-colored tumoral mass. When the overlapped green spheres cover the whole blue mass, the procedure is stopped. (**e**) After withdrawing the antenna, contrast-enhanced US is performed (*left*) and demonstrates an avascular volume of necrosis in the location of the mass. (**f**) Overlapping pretreatment CT over contrast-enhanced US in real time, it is seen that the volume of necrosis is definitely larger than the original tumor, as confirmed by contrast-enhanced CT acquired at 24 h after ablation (**g**)

able to clearly depict it, for its low conspicuity or for the presence of air or bone. In particular instances, when the target in invisible on US, once the target has been identified and marked on the virtual space and the device recognized by the system, it is possible to insert the device only under the control and tracking of the virtual navigation system. Of course, in this case the real-time US monitoring of the procedure is lacking. These systems can be particularly useful when procedures are performed in structures where US visibility is very poor or impossible, such as the lung or bone. Moreover, when a large tumor has to be ablated and multiple insertions of the device are needed, monitoring of the procedure with US is difficult or even impossible because gas develops and masks the area of treatment after the first insertion of the device. With virtual navigation it is possible to plan the treatment, knowing exactly which volume of ablation will be achieved with the device selected by the operator, overlaying to the volume to be treated several virtual ablative volumes. Thus, before starting the ablation, the operator is able to know how many insertions of the device will be needed and in which positions. Moreover, during treatment the operator can add a virtual ablated volume on the area of treatment, in order to recognize the area that has been already treated, even in presence of gas. Adding multiple virtual volumes of ablation, thanks to the constant visualization of the position of the virtual device, the operator can effectively treat the whole tumoral mass and create a sufficiently large peripheral safety halo (Fig. 10.5). Nowadays it is also technically possible to place a microsensor into an internal chamber created inside the device, in order for it to be as close as possible to the tip of the device itself. This may limit the problem of unforeseen needle bending. In classical needle-tracking systems with the sensor applied to the hub of the device, the position of the tip of the virtual device is estimated based on the location of the hub, so that, if the device deviates from the expected path due to the different stiffness of organs encountered (e.g., bones), the tip is represented on the virtual image in a position different from the real one. With dedicated needles and antennas with the sensor located in the inner chamber, this problem can be significantly reduced.

Respiratory motion can be a serious issue when image fusion and virtual navigation are used for moving organs, such as the liver, kidneys, or lung. In order to limit the misalignment of the real space with the virtual one, some methods can be employed. If ablation is performed under general anesthesia, high-frequency jet ventilation can be used to reduce respiratory motion: low-volume, fast rate ventilations are given to the patient, thus limiting lung excursions [11, 12]. More simply, when the respiratory phase in which the acquisition of image datasets has been achieved, co-registration and device insertion can be performed in the same respiratory phase, thus minimizing motion problems. Of course, this can be a very variable and unpredictable situation, as patients may alter their respiration for several reasons. Accordingly, a respiratory motion sensor can be applied to the patient's thorax to track his respiratory movements in real time. Thus, the operator can identify the best respiratory phase to perform the procedure, mark it on the respiration trace, and perform all the subsequent steps in the selected respiratory phase, automatically shown by the system [33, 52].

Immediately at the end of the ablative treatment, fusion imaging can be used to assess the result achieved. A new image dataset is acquired (e.g., contrast-enhanced US or CT) and fused with the pre-procedural image dataset (Fig. 10.5e). Thus, the volume of ablation achieved can be precisely overlapped on the pretreatment lesion volume in 3D by the operator (Fig. 10.5f). If the result achieved is not sufficiently large or not perfectly positioned in relation to the tumor location, an immediate re-treatment can be performed under the guidance of fusion imaging [3, 26, 29].

10.5 Clinical Applications of Fusion Imaging and Virtual Navigation in Interventional Procedures

Despite their significant advantages (greater precision, decrease of procedural time, difficult cases made easier), virtual navigation systems are not widely diffused yet, being generally considered expensive and complex to use. However, further technological advancements, reduction of costs, and increasing scientific evidence of efficacy will certainly lead to a greater diffusion in the near future.

In clinical practice, fusion imaging and virtual navigation have been mainly used for liver and kidney, for both biopsies and ablations [2, 4, 19, 20, 22, 26]. Biopsies of abdominal targets are generally performed under US guidance, but clinically there is an increasing need to target the most vital part of a mass, i.e., that with greater uptake on PET scan. Thus, fusion of PET and US or CT has been successfully used to target the most avid portion of tumors [13, 15, 64], and with the advancements of personalized medicine and molecular biology of tumors, fusion imaging and virtual navigation systems will play an increasingly important role. In the world of ablation, they are used to better identify and target inconspicuous or even sonographically undetectable liver or kidney tumors (Fig. 10.6). In a series of 295 liver tumors (162 HCCs and 133 metastases) that were undetectable with US, it was possible to achieve a correct tumor targeting in 282 of 295 (95.6 %) tumors using the guidance as an image fusion system (Virtual Navigation System, Esaote S.p.A., Genova, Italy) that combines real-time US with preacquired CT or MR images. This system is allowed for performing a successful treatment in the sonographic room using a

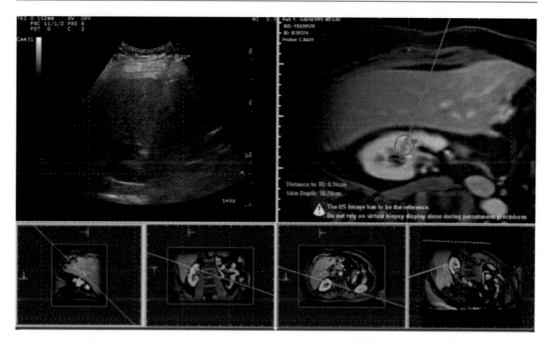

Fig. 10.6 Small (1 cm) renal tumor almost undetectable on US, but clearly showed on MRI, precisely targeted with real-time fusion of US and MRI after co-registration

simple, low-cost, widely available, and safe modality [26]. Krücker et al. [20] used the navigation assistance for performing ablations and biopsies of 51 lesions situated in various organs. They spent 5.8 ± 2.5 min of additional setup time for the navigation system and evaluated the mean fiducial registration error as 1.6 ± 0.7 mm. They concluded that the navigation system provided information unavailable using conventional guidance, with an increased successful completion of the procedure that was thought to be performed potentially more accurately, faster, with fewer CT scans, or greater operator confidence.

In the neck, when a US-guided biopsy or an ablation of a metastatic lymph node is planned and the identification of the pathological node is difficult or impossible with US, image fusion of US and PET scans and navigation can be successfully employed, as reported in recent literature [27, 30].

For interventional procedures of the lung and bones, CT is usually the guidance modality of first choice. Image fusion with precise tracking of the device can be added to conventional CT scans in order to reduce procedural time and radiation exposure (e.g., in young patients treated for osteoid osteomas) decreasing the number of CT scans needed [16–18, 35, 47]. Narsule et al. [35] compared lung procedures (biopsies and ablations) performed with and without an electromagnetic navigation system in 17 patients and reported a significantly lower time to perform lung ablations when using the navigation system. Grasso et al. [17] used a CT navigation system in 197 patients to perform lung biopsies. In comparison with a group of patients who underwent standard CT-guided lung biopsy, they found a significant reduction in procedure time, number of required CT scans, and radiation dose administered to patients in the group of patients in whom navigation system was used.

In the treatment of benign thyroid nodules, when several multiple device insertion and ablations are generally performed and gas formation strongly limits the visibility of the device, virtual navigation and needle tracking have been successfully used to monitor the procedure and have a clearer and faster assessment of the achieved volume of ablation, avoiding the need to wait for gas reabsorption [30, 59]. Turtulici et al. [59]

reported on the use of ultrasound-guided radio-frequency ablation of benign thyroid nodules assisted by a real-time virtual needle-tracking system in 45 patients. They concluded that this system could be useful in thyroid nodule ablation procedures because it is able to track the electrode tip even when it is obscured by the bubbles produced by the ablative process.

Conclusions

In conclusion, image fusion and virtual navigation represent an important advance for facilitating interventional procedures, being extremely helpful at all the procedural steps, from planning to targeting, through monitoring and follow-up thereby often enabling procedures that would otherwise be unfeasible using standard, single-modality image guidance. Moreover, these techniques can be extremely helpful for less experienced operators, increasing the confidence and shortening their learning curve. Accordingly, the increase in their utilization certainly holds the potential for expanding the number of cases suitable for minimally invasive image-guided procedures.

References

1. Abi-Jaoudeh N, Kruecker J, Kadoury S et al (2012) Multimodality image fusion-guided procedures: technique, accuracy, and applications. Cardiovasc Intervent Radiol 35:986–998. doi:10.1007/s00270-012-0446-5
2. Amalou H, Wood BJ (2012) Multimodality fusion with MRI, CT, and ultrasound contrast for ablation of renal cell carcinoma. Case Rep Urol 2012:390912. doi:10.1155/2012/390912
3. Appelbaum L, Mahgerefteh SY, Sosna J, Goldberg SN (2013) Image-guided fusion and navigation: applications in tumor ablation. Tech Vasc Interv Radiol 16:287–295. doi:10.1053/j.tvir.2013.08.011
4. Appelbaum L, Solbiati L, Sosna J et al (2013) Evaluation of an electromagnetic image-fusion navigation system for biopsy of small lesions: assessment of accuracy in an in vivo swine model. Acad Radiol 20:209–217. doi:10.1016/j.acra.2012.09.020
5. Baulch J, Gandhi M, Sommerville J, Panizza B (2015) 3T MRI evaluation of large nerve perineural spread of head and neck cancers. J Med Imaging Radiat Oncol. doi:10.1111/1754-9485.12338
6. Baumgart DC, Müller HP, Grittner U et al (2015) US-based real-time elastography for the detection of fibrotic gut tissue in patients with stricturing Crohn disease. Radiology 275:889–899. doi:10.1148/radiol.14141929
7. Belli A-M, Markose G, Morgan R (2012) The role of interventional radiology in the management of abdominal visceral artery aneurysms. Cardiovasc Intervent Radiol 35:234–243. doi:10.1007/s00270-011-0201-3
8. Beyer T, Townsend DW, Brun T et al (2000) A combined PET/CT scanner for clinical oncology. J Nucl Med 41:1369–1379
9. Sconfienza LM1, Mauri G, Grossi F, et al (2013) Pleural and peripheral lung lesions: comparison of US- and CT-guided biopsy. Radiology 266(3):930–935. doi:10.1148/radiol.12112077
10. Chen MY, Shanbhag SM, Arai AE (2013) Submillisievert median radiation dose for coronary angiography with a second-generation 320-detector row CT scanner in 107 consecutive patients. Radiology 267:76–85. doi:10.1148/radiol.13122621
11. Chung DYF, Tse DML, Boardman P et al (2014) High-frequency jet ventilation under general anesthesia facilitates CT-guided lung tumor thermal ablation compared with normal respiration under conscious analgesic sedation. J Vasc Interv Radiol 25:1463–1469. doi:10.1016/j.jvir.2014.02.026
12. Denys A, Lachenal Y, Duran R et al (2014) Use of high-frequency jet ventilation for percutaneous tumor ablation. Cardiovasc Intervent Radiol 37:140–146. doi:10.1007/s00270-013-0620-4
13. Di Mauro E, Solbiati M, De Beni S et al (2013) Virtual navigator real-time ultrasound fusion imaging with positron emission tomography for liver interventions. Conf Proc IEEE Eng Med Biol Soc 2013:1406–1409. doi:10.1109/EMBC.2013.6609773
14. Eisenberg JD, Gervais DA, Singh S et al (2015) Radiation exposure from CT-guided ablation of renal masses: effects on life expectancy. AJR Am J Roentgenol 204:335–342. doi:10.2214/AJR.14.13010
15. Giesel FL, Mehndiratta A, Locklin J et al (2009) Image fusion using CT, MRI and PET for treatment planning, navigation and follow up in percutaneous RFA. Exp Oncol 31:106–114
16. Grasso RF, Cazzato RL, Luppi G et al (2013) Percutaneous lung biopsies: performance of an optical CT-based navigation system with a low-dose protocol. Eur Radiol 23:3071–3076. doi:10.1007/s00330-013-2932-9
17. Grasso RF, Faiella E, Luppi G et al (2013) Percutaneous lung biopsy: comparison between an augmented reality CT navigation system and standard CT-guided technique. Int J Comput Assist Radiol Surg 8:837–848. doi:10.1007/s11548-013-0816-8
18. Hakime A, Deschamps F, De Carvalho EGM et al (2011) Clinical evaluation of spatial accuracy of a fusion imaging technique combining previously acquired computed tomography and real-time ultrasound for imaging of liver metastases. Cardiovasc

Intervent Radiol 34:338–344. doi:10.1007/s00270-010-9979-7

19. Hung AJ, Ma Y, Zehnder P et al (2012) Percutaneous radiofrequency ablation of virtual tumours in canine kidney using Global Positioning System-like technology. BJU Int 109:1398–1403. doi:10.1111/j.1464-410X.2011.10648.x

20. Krücker J, Xu S, Venkatesan A et al (2011) Clinical utility of real-time fusion guidance for biopsy and ablation. J Vasc Interv Radiol 22:515–524. doi:10.1016/j.jvir.2010.10.033

21. Lell MM, Wildberger JE, Alkadhi H et al (2015) Evolution in computed tomography: the battle for speed and dose. Invest Radiol. doi:10.1097/RLI.0000000000000172

22. Liu F-Y, Yu X-L, Liang P et al (2012) Microwave ablation assisted by a real-time virtual navigation system for hepatocellular carcinoma undetectable by conventional ultrasonography. Eur J Radiol 81:1455–1459. doi:10.1016/j.ejrad.2011.03.057

23. Livraghi T, Solbiati L, Meloni F et al (2003) Percutaneous radiofrequency ablation of liver metastases in potential candidates for resection: the "test-of-time approach". Cancer 97:3027–3035. doi:10.1002/cncr.11426

24. Lu Q, Cao W, Huang L et al (2012) CT-guided percutaneous microwave ablation of pulmonary malignancies: Results in 69 cases. World J Surg Oncol 10:80. doi:10.1186/1477-7819-10-80

25. Mauri G, De Beni S, Forzoni L et al (2014) Virtual navigator automatic registration technology in abdominal application. Conf Proc IEEE Eng Med Biol Soc 2014:5570–5574

26. Mauri G, Cova L, De Beni S et al (2014) Real-time US-CT/MRI image fusion for guidance of thermal ablation of liver tumors undetectable with US: results in 295 cases. Cardiovasc Intervent Radiol. doi:10.1007/s00270-014-0897-y

27. Mauri G, Cova L, Tondolo T et al (2013) Percutaneous laser ablation of metastatic lymph nodes in the neck from papillary thyroid carcinoma: preliminary results. J Clin Endocrinol Metab 98:E1203–E1207. doi:10.1210/jc.2013-1140

28. Mauri G, Mattiuz C, Sconfienza LM et al (2014) Role of interventional radiology in the management of complications after pancreatic surgery: a pictorial review. Insights Imaging. doi:10.1007/s13244-014-0372-y

29. Mauri G, Porazzi E, Cova L et al (2014) Intraprocedural contrast-enhanced ultrasound (CEUS) in liver percutaneous radiofrequency ablation: clinical impact and health technology assessment. Insights Imaging 5:209–216. doi:10.1007/s13244-014-0315-7

30. Mauri G, Solbiati L (2015) Virtual navigation and fusion imaging in percutaneous ablations in the neck. Ultrasound Med Biol 41:898. doi:10.1016/j.ultrasmedbio.2014.10.022

31. Miwa K, Matsuo M, Ogawa S et al (2014) Re-irradiation of recurrent glioblastoma multiforme using 11C-methionine PET/CT/MRI image fusion for hypofractionated stereotactic radiotherapy by intensity modulated radiation therapy. Radiat Oncol 9:181. doi:10.1186/1748-717X-9-181

32. Molla N, AlMenieir N, Simoneau E et al (2014) The role of interventional radiology in the management of hepatocellular carcinoma. Curr Oncol 21:e480–e492. doi:10.3747/co.21.1829

33. Muller A, Petrusca L, Auboiroux V et al (2013) Management of respiratory motion in extracorporeal high-intensity focused ultrasound treatment in upper abdominal organs: current status and perspectives. Cardiovasc Intervent Radiol 36:1464–1476. doi:10.1007/s00270-013-0713-0

34. Nagamachi S, Nishii R, Wakamatsu H et al (2013) The usefulness of (18)F-FDG PET/MRI fusion image in diagnosing pancreatic tumor: comparison with (18)F-FDG PET/CT. Ann Nucl Med 27:554–563. doi:10.1007/s12149-013-0719-3

35. Narsule CK, Sales Dos Santos R, Gupta A et al (2012) The efficacy of electromagnetic navigation to assist with computed tomography-guided percutaneous thermal ablation of lung tumors. Innovations (Phila) 7:187–190. doi:10.1097/IMI.0b013e318265b127

36. Oriuchi N, Higuchi T, Ishikita T et al (2006) Present role and future prospects of positron emission tomography in clinical oncology. Cancer Sci 97:1291–1297. doi:10.1111/j.1349-7006.2006.00341.x

37. Oto A, Sethi I, Karczmar G et al (2013) MR imaging-guided focal laser ablation for prostate cancer: phase I trial. Radiology 267:932–940. doi:10.1148/radiol.13121652

38. Pacella CM, Bizzarri G, Spiezia S et al (2004) Thyroid tissue: US-guided percutaneous laser thermal ablation. Radiology 232:272–280. doi:10.1148/radiol.2321021368

39. Paparo F, Piccardo A, Bacigalupo L et al (2015) Multimodality fusion imaging in abdominal and pelvic malignancies: current applications and future perspectives. Abdom Imaging. doi:10.1007/s00261-015-0435-7

40. Paparo F, Piccardo A, Bacigalupo L et al (2015) Multimodality fusion imaging in abdominal and pelvic malignancies: current applications and future perspectives. Abdom Imaging. doi:10.1007/s00261-015-0435-7

41. Paparo F, Piccazzo R, Cevasco L et al (2014) Advantages of percutaneous abdominal biopsy under PET-CT/ultrasound fusion imaging guidance: a pictorial essay. Abdom Imaging 39:1102–1113. doi:10.1007/s00261-014-0143-8

42. Prada F, Del Bene M, Mattei L et al (2015) Preoperative magnetic resonance and intraoperative ultrasound fusion imaging for real-time neuronavigation in brain tumor surgery. Ultraschall Med 36:174–186. doi:10.1055/s-0034-1385347

43. Price SJ, Young AMH, Scotton WJ et al (2015) Multimodal MRI can identify perfusion and metabolic changes in the invasive margin of glioblastomas. J Magn Reson Imaging. doi:10.1002/jmri.24996

44. Quinn SF, Murtagh FR, Chatfield R, Kori SH (1988) CT-guided nerve root block and ablation. AJR Am J Roentgenol 151:1213–1216. doi:10.2214/ajr.151.6.1213

45. Rehnitz C, Sprengel SD, Lehner B et al (2012) CT-guided radiofrequency ablation of osteoid osteoma and osteoblastoma: clinical success and long-term follow up in 77 patients. Eur J Radiol 81:3426–3434. doi:10.1016/j.ejrad.2012.04.037

46. Rempp H, Waibel L, Hoffmann R et al (2012) MR-guided radiofrequency ablation using a wide-bore 1.5-T MR system: clinical results of 213 treated liver lesions. Eur Radiol 22:1972–1982. doi:10.1007/s00330-012-2438-x

47. Santos RS, Gupta A, Ebright MI et al (2010) Electromagnetic navigation to aid radiofrequency ablation and biopsy of lung tumors. Ann Thorac Surg 89:265–268. doi:10.1016/j.athoracsur.2009.06.006

48. Sconfienza LM, Mauri G, Grossi F et al (2013) Pleural and peripheral lung lesions: comparison of US- and CT-guided biopsy. Radiology 266:930–935. doi:10.1148/radiol.12112077

49. Shyn PB (2013) Interventional positron emission tomography/computed tomography: state-of-the-art. Tech Vasc Interv Radiol 16:182–190. doi:10.1053/j.tvir.2013.02.014

50. Shyn PB, Mauri G, Alencar RO et al (2014) Percutaneous imaging-guided cryoablation of liver tumors: predicting local progression on 24-hour MRI. AJR Am J Roentgenol 203:1–11. doi:10.2214/AJR.13.10747

51. Shyn PB, Tatli S, Sahni VA et al (2014) PET/CT-guided percutaneous liver mass biopsies and ablations: targeting accuracy of a single 20 s breath-hold PET acquisition. Clin Radiol 69:410–415. doi:10.1016/j.crad.2013.11.013

52. Shyn PB, Tatli S, Sainani NI et al (2011) Minimizing image misregistration during PET/CT-guided percutaneous interventions with monitored breath-hold PET and CT acquisitions. J Vasc Interv Radiol 22:1287–1292. doi:10.1016/j.jvir.2011.06.015

53. Silverman SG, Tuncali K, Morrison PR (2005) MR Imaging-guided percutaneous tumor ablation. Acad Radiol 12:1100–1109. doi:10.1016/j.acra.2005.05.019

54. Solbiati L, Ahmed M, Cova L et al (2012) Small liver colorectal metastases treated with percutaneous radiofrequency ablation: local response rate and long-term survival with up to 10-year follow-up. Radiology 265:958–968. doi:10.1148/radiol.12111851

55. Solbiati L, Giangrande A, De Pra L et al (1985) Percutaneous ethanol injection of parathyroid tumors under US guidance: treatment for secondary hyperparathyroidism. Radiology 155:607–610. doi:10.1148/radiology.155.3.3889999

56. Solbiati L, Ierace T, Tonolini M, Cova L (2004) Guidance and monitoring of radiofrequency liver tumor ablation with contrast-enhanced ultrasound. Eur J Radiol 51(Suppl):S19–S23

57. Takeshita J, Masago K, Kato R et al (2015) CT-guided fine-needle aspiration and core needle biopsies of pulmonary lesions: a single-center experience with 750 biopsies in Japan. AJR Am J Roentgenol 204:29–34. doi:10.2214/AJR.14.13151

58. Tatli S, Gerbaudo VH, Mamede M et al (2010) Abdominal masses sampled at PET/CT-guided percutaneous biopsy: initial experience with registration of prior PET/CT images. Radiology 256:305–311. doi:10.1148/radiol.10090931

59. Turtulici G, Orlandi D, Corazza A et al (2014) Percutaneous radiofrequency ablation of benign thyroid nodules assisted by a virtual needle tracking system. Ultrasound Med Biol 40:1447–1452. doi:10.1016/j.ultrasmedbio.2014.02.017

60. Venkatesan AM, Kadoury S, Abi-Jaoudeh N et al (2011) Real-time FDG PET guidance during biopsies and radiofrequency ablation using multimodality fusion with electromagnetic navigation. Radiology 260:848–856. doi:10.1148/radiol.11101985

61. Wallach D, Toporek G, Weber S et al (2014) Comparison of freehand-navigated and aiming device-navigated targeting of liver lesions. Int J Med Robot 10:35–43. doi:10.1002/rcs.1505

62. Wood BJ, Locklin JK, Viswanathan A et al (2007) Technologies for guidance of radiofrequency ablation in the multimodality interventional suite of the future. J Vasc Interv Radiol 18:9–24. doi:10.1016/j.jvir.2006.10.013

63. Wu H, Wilkins LR, Ziats NP et al (2014) Real-time monitoring of radiofrequency ablation and postablation assessment: accuracy of contrast-enhanced US in experimental rat liver model. Radiology 270:107–116. doi:10.1148/radiol.13121999

64. Zaidi H, Montandon M-L, Alavi A (2010) The clinical role of fusion imaging using PET, CT, and MR imaging. Magn Reson Imaging Clin N Am 18:133–149. doi:10.1016/j.mric.2009.09.010

Navigable Ultrasound, 3D Ultrasound and Fusion Imaging in Neurosurgery

11

Aliasgar V. Moiyadi and Geirmund Unsgård

11.1 Concept of Navigation

Navigation, as the term connotes in general usage, implies the ability to be led or guided along a particular route to a specific location. This assumes even greater importance in neurosurgical procedures where access is usually restricted, targets often deep seated hidden away from obvious view and the trajectory to the target literally a minefield (of eloquent neural tissue) where one wrong step could lead to devastating consequences. Navigation provides a virtual road map allowing the neurosurgeon to plan and rehearse the actual procedure, selecting the most optimal strategy before executing it. Conventional navigation typically uses preoperatively acquired MR (and less frequently CT) images of the patient which are then projected onto the actual physical space of the patient itself by a procedure called image-to-patient registration. This process

A.V. Moiyadi, MCh (✉)
Neurosurgery Services, Department of Surgical Oncology, Tata Memorial Centre and Advanced Centre for Treatment Research and Education in Cancer (ACTREC), 1221, HBB, E Borges Road, Parel, Mumbai 400012, India
e-mail: aliasgar.moiyadi@gmail.com

G. Unsgård, MD, PhD
Neurosurgical Department, St Olav University Hospital and Norwegian University of Science and Technology, Trondheim, Norway
e-mail: geirmund.unsgard@ntnu.no

of registration ensures that the virtual image space (as in the MR) is accurately matched to the patient's physical space (as at the time of the surgery) allowing the neurosurgeon to visualize the surgical space in terms of the MR images and look (virtually) beyond the visible anatomy seen in the operative field. As is obvious, a lot of computational methodology is essential for ensuring accurate navigation. At the heart of navigation technology is the ability to faithfully track instruments and tools within the physical space and project this onto the image space, permitting the user to get the "bearings" right at various time points during the procedure. Neuronavigation or image-guided surgery which was introduced into routine neurosurgical practice in the 1990s revolutionized the way neurosurgical procedures were planned and executed especially with regard to intra-axial tumour surgery [58, 59]. Despite the early enthusiasm, it soon became evident that changes in intraoperative anatomical space during the surgical procedure would not reflect dynamically in the preoperatively acquired (and hence unchanged) MR images – the so-called phenomenon of "brain shift" [1, 33, 35]. It was clear that to remain continually accurate (and hence relevant and useful) during the entire surgical procedure, updating the images to reflect the continuously changing intracranial anatomy dynamically was essential. This paved the way for the introduction of intraoperative imaging. Though intraoperative MR remains the so-called

F. Prada et al. (eds.), *Intraoperative Ultrasound (IOUS) in Neurosurgery:*
From Standard B-mode to Elastosonography, DOI 10.1007/978-3-319-25268-1_11

gold standard, logistical challenges (including cost, time and resource utilization) make it difficult to implement except in a handful of centres globally. The intraoperative ultrasound (IOUS) which was actually used as an intraoperative imaging tool much before the MR was (see chapter on history) is a useful alternative. Combining the IOUS with navigational technology provides a synergistic benefit allowing reliable real-time image guidance.

11.2　Navigated Ultrasound

Navigated US is basically "tracked" US images. At the heart of the navigated ultrasound is the probe calibration. Probe calibration renders the US navigable. Once the probe is calibrated and tracked, the US volume can be projected onto the actual anatomical space of the patient. This process can be imagined to be similar to the image-to-patient registration in conventional navigation systems whereby MR images are "registered" to the patient during navigation. However, as the US images are acquired within the same 3D space in which the navigation is being performed (with a common reference frame), there is no registration inaccuracy (unlike preoperative MR-/CT-based navigation where it is inherent). Various probe calibration strategies are utilized for this purpose [22, 27, 37]. Using the various calibration techniques, independent stand-alone US probes (sector as well as linear probes) can be manually calibrated and integrated into navigation systems [6, 17, 50]. Most of the calibration solutions are specific to the probe being used, often making the procedure complicated if multiple probes are to be used. Newer techniques of calibration can overcome some of these limitations [3]. Some commercial systems are available which utilize precalibrated and integrated US probes [13]. This enhances the ease of use, much like a plug and play device.

Advantages of navigated US: Tracking of the US enables the images to be defined in a particular 3D space of reference. When this 3D space is coregistered with the patient, the US images can be superimposed onto the patient anatomy and pro-

vide real-time guidance. Further, using calibrated tools (instruments coregistered to the same reference frame of the 3D space), the surgeon can work within the navigated US images, constantly being guided with respect to the actual position of the instruments. Most importantly, coregistration with preoperative images (using the common frame of reference) allows correlation of the US and preoperative MR images, providing the so-called image guidance for the US itself [29] (Fig. 11.1).

Many groups have described coregistration of 2DUS with navigation to obtain navigable 2DUS [7, 11, 14, 18]. Though early reports described two-platform solutions (where the navigation unit and ultrasound scanner are physically two separate units), most contemporary reports employ a single-platform solution, thereby improving ergonomics and the overall accuracy of the device [50, 56]. The planar 2DUS image is co-displayed along with the corresponding MR image (either side by side or as an overlay technique). Renovanz et al. compared 2DUS with navigated 2DUS for resection of gliomas and concluded that the navigated US offers better image resolution and improves orientation within the surgical field [42]. They however could not see any improved benefit in the overall extent of resection using navigated US. Miller et al. also reported their experience with navigated 2DUS [29]. Whereas they did not find NUS to improve the image quality, the co-display with MR images helped interpret artefacts better and delineate tumour boundaries more reliably. Most importantly, the NUS helped orientation by depicting the relevant planar anatomy (in the MR image) beyond the field of view of the US image itself. However, there are limitations with using navigated 2DUS. When only 2DUS images are navigated, the orientation problem may still persist if the plane of insonation is not a conventional, easy to understand plane (axial, coronal or sagittal). Also when multiple 2DUS scans are taken serially and need to be compared, it becomes difficult if they are noncoplanar (Fig. 11.3). Use of navigated 3DUS overcomes this limitation [2, 19, 51, 56]. The 3D volume can be displayed in any desired plane, and these can be compared reliably over serial acquisitions. Using navigated 3DUS,

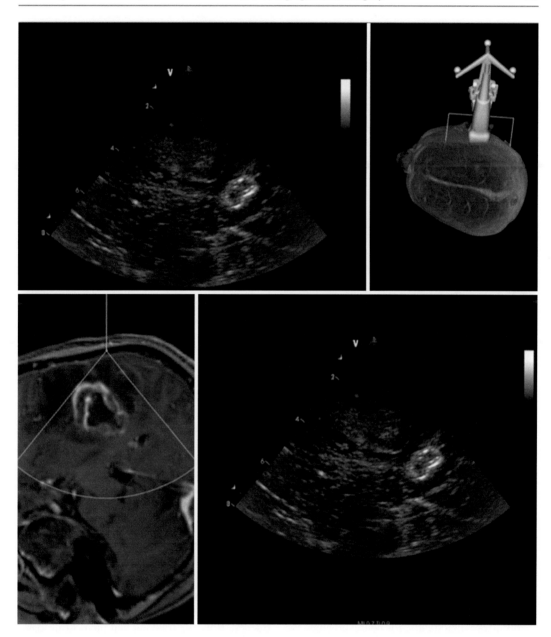

Fig. 11.1 Advantages of image-guided navigable 2D ultrasound. *Upper row* shows the planar 2D ultrasound image of a glioma. Though the lesion is well appreciated, it is difficult to orient the lesion within the brain. *Lower row* shows the same 2DUS image co-displayed along with the corresponding MR plane, allowing better overview and orientation of the entire 3D space

it is also possible to calculate and correct for brain shift in all three planes (see next section) (Figs. 11.2 and 11.3).

A significant limitation of any US (2D or 3D) presently remains the inability to obtain a large volume field of view. Neurosurgeons being accustomed to the full head views of MRI often find this unsettling. Using spatial summation of multiple 3DUS views, Ji et al. reported increasing the overall field of view of 3DUS [15]. However, the orientation problem may still not be completely overcome. Using image fusion, it is

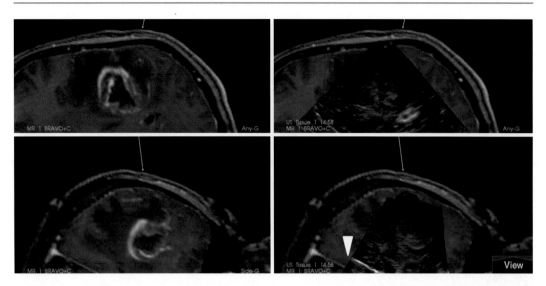

Fig. 11.2 Navigated 3D ultrasound. 3D ultrasound allows multiplanar representation of the insonated lesion. Right panel shows the same lesion in Fig. 11.1 as seen with a 3DUS acquisition. Two orthogonal planes can be simultaneously depicted (*upper and lower rows*). The images can be overlaid (*right panel*) or co-displayed (*left panel*) with the corresponding MR images to provide better 3D orientation. Note the brain shift in the right lower panel (*white arrowhead*) evident in the discordance between the falx as seen on the MR and the corresponding US image

possible to combine information from MR and US – thus extracting the best of both – US for real-time update and MR for full head view and anatomical detail.

11.3 Three-Dimensional Ultrasound (3DUS)

What is it: 3D ultrasound basically is volumetric ultrasound data, very similar to how conventional CT and MR scans are acquired. Once acquired, the 3D volume can then be used to provide multiplanar images according to the end user's requirements. More importantly, for neurosurgeons, the acquired data can be sliced into conventional axial, coronal and sagittal planes for ease of understanding.

How is it obtained: 3DUS data is generated by summation of multiple 2DUS images. Most often, this is done by moving a conventional 2DUS probe over the field of interest, thereby generating a series of 2DUS images which are then reconstructed to produce a 3D volume. Though the quality of the 2DUS probe is crucial for the 3DUS volume quality, the method of image transfer and processing is also very important. Some systems utilize the analogue video source from the US machine which is subsequently digitized for further post-processing [51]. Better image quality may be obtained by using digital video transfer of the source US images [47]. Once imported, the US data is then reconstructed using various algorithms [30, 48]. The algorithms used, though important, are less essential for the overall image quality eventually than the type of source data used [47]. Regardless of the source images used and the method of post-processing, reconstruction of 2DUS image stacks into 3DUS requires the probe to be tracked. Both the tracking and the post-processing used introduce a small but finite error into the overall accuracy of the system [20]. If the freehand 2DUS acquisition has been suboptimal, "holes" or gaps may be found in the reconstructed 3DUS volume and could hamper eventual clinical application. Motorized 3DUS probes eliminate these inaccuracies and limitations by acquiring a 3DUS in real time. The need to reconstruct images into a 3D volume is eliminated and better image quality may be obtained [4, 32]. Whereas the 3DUS volume produced by

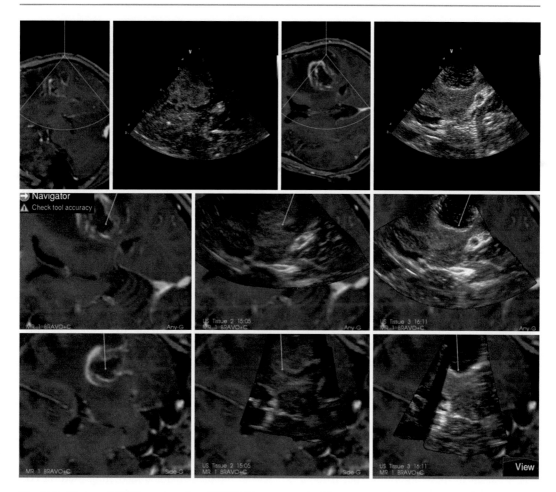

Fig. 11.3 Navigated 2DUS versus navigated 3DUS. Upper row shows two serially acquired navigated 2DUS images before (*left*) and after (*right*) resection. Note that the two images are noncoplanar (as evident from the MRI overlay in each image). Lower row shows the same information as acquired by a navigated 3DUS. Orthogonal images of the pre-resection (*centre*) and post-resection (*right*) scans can be displayed (*upper* and *lower panels* of the *lower row* image) in the same plane allowing for meaningful comparison of the images serially

such probes can be generated without the need for navigation or probe tracking, such tracking is desirable if the 3D volume is to be used for the purpose of navigation during the surgery.

11.4 Intermodality (MR and US) Fusion and Brain Shift Correction

One of the main limitations of US is the lack of orientation. Absence of a full head view can lead of difficulties in intuitively identifying the pre-

cise anatomical region depicted by the US. This may be particularly disconcerting for beginners, unaccustomed to US image interpretation. An effective solution is image coregistration of the US with corresponding MR images as has been discussed in the previous section. This is now possible and widely available. This image coregistration however loses its utility once there is brain shift and deformation. Re-registering the updated US with MRI using various algorithms for correcting the brain shift allows updating the MR images repeatedly and permits the continual use of the MR for navigation. This "image fusion" can be achieved in many ways [14, 16, 34, 36, 39, 43, 52]. The various algorithms used take into account coregistration inaccuracies as well as brain shift modelling and correction. Point-based or surface-matching-based techniques are routinely used in registration of preoperative MR data to patient space in conventional navigation. Using the same principles, intermodality image-to-image fusion can be obtained utilizing common, known anatomical landmarks in the different sets of images (US and MR). Examples include matching blood vessels or midline structures [41, 49]. However, this requires manual intervention during surgery, may be error prone and is very difficult to automate [8]. Another method for reliable image-to-image fusion is the voxel-based technique using maximization of mutual information [23, 24, 57] for intermodal image fusion. However this may be difficult for MR-US fusion because of inherent differences in MR and US image composition. Another rigid body model is the block matching technique suggested by Chalopin et al. [5]. Mercier et al. describe a "pseudo-ultrasound" approach to transform MR images for registration with corresponding US images [26]. However, the rigid body affine transformations that are used in these algorithms fail if there is inelastic deformation, as is the case during tumour resection in the brain. To incorporate the inelastic deformation, other computational techniques have been used such as a finite element biomechanical model [10] and a viscous fluid model [8]. However, these are complex and difficult to integrate on a real-time basis.

Brain shift correction and image fusion are most accurate before the start of tumour resection when the deformation is more likely to be elastic (uniform in all directions). With progressive tumour resection, algorithms become more complex because the deformation becomes inelastic (variable in different directions three-dimensionally) and hence fusion less reliable [39].

Whereas most of the fusion strategies aim to correct the MR based on the US, some prefer enhancing the US based on the MR. Chalopin et al. describe a fusion technique that facilitates modulation of the US images to sharpen their borders and "fill in" missing details [5]. This is based on a "block matching" technique using tumour segmentation of the preoperative MRI to match with the US image. The resultant-improved US image resolution can be reliably used for delineation of tumour boundaries.

Besides the advantage of improving orientation and permitting brain shift correction, image fusion techniques can be used to identify ultrasonically invisible targets using real-time intraoperative ultrasound fused with preoperative MR (when the target is visible on the MR but not the US) [9]. Moreover, image fusion can help complement the utility of the US by providing information that cannot be obtained from US images, such as functional information. Fusing preoperative fMRI and DTI data with the US combines real-time anatomical information provided by the US with functional information from the MRI [40].

Regardless of the type of fusion technique employed, all strategies aim to fuse the US (which is updated in real time but may lack complete anatomical information) with MR (which has more complete and "panoramic" details but lacks real-time updates) and get the best of both worlds. However, accuracy and reliability of the fusion are always questionable because regardless of the mathematical modelling used for correction, it is almost impossible to predict the three-dimensional nature of the shift in real time. Hence though a general orientation may be obtained, to assess residual tumour, it is best to rely only on the updated US image [39].

11.5 Stand-Alone Navigated Ultrasound

Despite all efforts to improve the accuracy of MR-US fusion, errors persist. Further, the actual potential and advantage of the US (its ability to provide real-time information in quick time) may be underexploited. This has spurred interest in the use of US directly as the sole means of intraoperative navigation [54]. Miller et al. reported use of direct navigable US in two cases where conventional navigation failed [28]. In both cases, the US was sufficient for fruitful completion of the planned procedure. In a larger study of 18 cases, it was reported that direct 3D navigated US was useful in intraoperative navigation without the need for preoperative MR-based navigation [38]. The authors found the 3DUS adequate for visualization of the target lesion and achieving the goal of resection in the gliomas. Whereas in both these reports, the US was used as a stand-alone adjunct due to failure of the conventional navigation, it has been our own experience (unpublished observations) that surgery can proceed very well with the US only, provided a good quality optimal 3D scan is obtained. The learning curve is pretty steep and can be quickly overcome. It helps when overlay of MRI is available (at least during the early part of the neurosurgeon's clinical experience), but it is not mandatory. Serial acquisition of US images during the course of resection allows for a dynamic control on the resection process, assessing the residue while eliminating artefacts [46]. Use of US-to-US image fusion strategies may help improve detection of residual tumour and track the progress of surgery incorporating brain shift correction in real time [26]. Using stand-alone 3DUS obviates the need for a dedi-cated preoperative MR (which adds to cost and in some situations such as emergencies is not possible). This could be a considerable advantage in busy departments especially in resource-constrained settings where the navigable 3DUS could be a cost-effective alternative to intraoperative MR (Fig. 11.4).

11.6 Clinical Utility of Navigated Ultrasound

The clinical utility of navigated US has been amply demonstrated. Integrating 3DUS (whether it is reconstructed or real-time 3DUS) into navigation is very useful for intraoperative guidance [51]. This has been described for resection control in intra-axial low-grade as well as high-grade gliomas [6, 19, 31, 55]. Low-grade gliomas are better demarcated with a linear array probe than a phased array probe (Fig. 11.5). With a linear array probe and a high-end scanner, the low-grade glioma tissue can be gradually removed towards the borders (Fig. 11.6). Navigated 3DUS has been shown to improve resection rates in

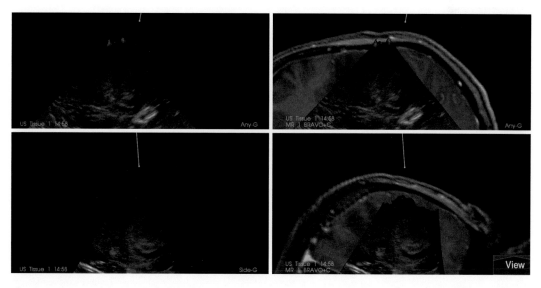

Fig. 11.4 Direct stand-alone navigable 3DUS. Screenshot from the navigation system showing the same lesion as in Fig. 11.2. In this case the direct navigable 3DUS function was used (as seen in the *left panel*) providing excellent multiplanar (biplanar in this case as dual any plane view was selected) images. Corresponding MR overlay is seen on the right panel. This however can be dispensed with if it is not available or not required or inaccurate (loss of registration or brain shift)

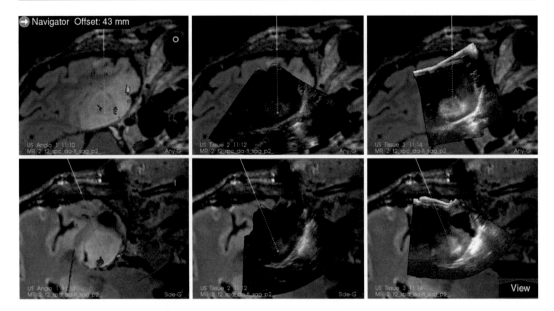

Fig. 11.5 Snapshot of the monitor during operation of low-grade glioma (*upper row* is a plane close to an axial plane, and *lower row* is a plane 90 ° to the former plane through the virtual line of the navigator). The images are cross sections from 3D MR flair with overlay of corresponding 3DUS cross sections. To the *left*: 3DUS angiography (power Doppler). In the *middle*: 3DUS tissue acquired with a 8 MHz-phased array probe. To the *right*: 3DUS acquired with a 12 Mhz linear array probe. The 8 MHz-phased array probe shows only the central part of the tumour, probably the part with highest cell density

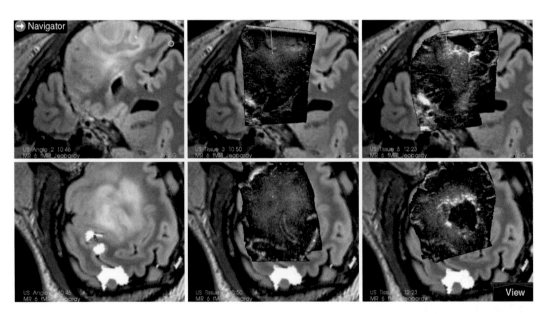

Fig. 11.6 Snapshot of the navigation monitor during resection of a low-grade glioma showing 3DUS in the beginning of the resection (*middle column*) and after some removal (*right column*). The *lower row* shows the tip view which is a plane perpendicular to the navigator line through the tip

gliomas permitting more radical resections. It is well known that extent of resection is an important prognostic factor in survival in both low- and high-grade gliomas. Though there is presently no direct evidence supporting the role of US-guided resections in improving survival (unlike level I evidence for IOMR or ALA-guided resections), the inference can be extrapolated from the numerous studies describing its benefits in obtaining radical resections. Saether et al. also report that compared to historical cohorts, use of 3DUS in their experience improved survival in patients with glioblastomas [45]. In our hands too, use of navigated 3DUS has shown to be independently associated with improved survival in glioblastomas (Moiyadi et al. unpublished data).

Besides resection control of gliomas, navigated ultrasound can be used for guiding resection of many other masses as well as vascular lesions. Intraoperative Doppler angiography is particularly of benefit providing updated vascular anatomy and guiding surgeries for AVMs and vascular lesions [12, 21, 25, 44, 53, 60]. The scope of application of the US is only limited practically by its ability to insonate a particular lesion. Therefore, almost any lesion (neoplastic as well as non-neoplastic) can be visualized using the US.

Conclusions

Navigated ultrasound and 3D ultrasound overcome the significant limitations of conventional 2D ultrasound. Multimodal image fusion permits combination of imaging modalities to extract maximum information and complement the individual modalities themselves. Clinical utility of this technology is established and could be a very effective tool during intracranial surgery.

References

1. Arbel T, Morandi X, Comeau RM, Collins DL. Automatic non-linear MRI-ultrasound registration for the correction of intra-operative brain deformations. Comput Aided Surg. 2004;9(4):123–36.

2. Becker G, Hofmann E, Woydt M, Hulsmann U, Maurer M, Lindner A, Becker T, Krone A. Postoperative neuroimaging of high-grade gliomas: comparison of transcranial sonography, magnetic resonance imaging, and computed tomography. Neurosurgery. 1999;44(3):469–77; discussion 477–468.

3. Bo LE, Hofstad EF, Lindseth F, Hernes TA. Versatile robotic probe calibration for position tracking in ultrasound imaging. Phys Med Biol. 2015;60(9):3499–513.

4. Bozinov O, Burkhardt JK, Fischer CM, Kockro RA, Bernays RL, Bertalanffy H. Advantages and limitations of intraoperative 3D ultrasound in neurosurgery. Technical note. Acta Neurochir Suppl. 2011;109:191–6.

5. Chalopin C, Lindenberg R, Arlt F, Müns A, Meixensberger J, Lindner D (2012) Brain tumor enhancement revealed by 3D intraoperative ultrasound imaging in a navigation system. Biomed Eng 57(SI-1 Track-B)

6. Coburger J, Konig RW, Scheuerle A, Engelke J, Hlavac M, Thal DR, Wirtz CR. Navigated high frequency ultrasound: description of technique and clinical comparison with conventional intracranial ultrasound. World Neurosurg. 2014;82(3–4):366–75.

7. Comeau RM, Fenster A, Peters TM. Intraoperative US in interactive image-guided neurosurgery. Radiographics. 1998;18(4):1019–27.

8. D'Agostino E, Maes F, Vandermeulen D, Suetens P. A viscous fluid model for multimodal non-rigid image registration using mutual information. Med Image Anal. 2003;7(4):565–75.

9. Ewertsen C, Grossjohann HS, Nielsen KR, Torp-Pedersen S, Nielsen MB. Biopsy guided by real-time sonography fused with MRI: a phantom study. AJR Am J Roentgenol. 2008;190(6):1671–4.

10. Ferrant M, Nabavi A, Macq B, Jolesz FA, Kikinis R, Warfield SK. Registration of 3-D intraoperative MR images of the brain using a finite-element biomechanical model. IEEE Trans Med Imaging. 2001;20(12):1384–97.

11. Giorgi C, Casolino DS. Preliminary clinical experience with intraoperative stereotactic ultrasound imaging. Stereotact Funct Neurosurg. 1997;68(1–4 Pt 1):54–8.

12. Glasker S, Shah MJ, Hippchen B, Neumann HP, van Velthoven V. Doppler-sonographically guided resection of central nervous system hemangioblastomas. Neurosurgery. 2011;68(2 Suppl Operative):267–75; discussion 274–265.

13. Gronningsaeter A, Kleven A, Ommedal S, Aarseth TE, Lie T, Lindseth F, Lango T, Unsgard G. SonoWand, an ultrasound-based neuronavigation system. Neurosurgery. 2000;47(6):1373–9; discussion 1379–1380.

14. Hata N, Dohi T, Iseki H, Takakura K. Development of a frameless and armless stereotactic neuronavigation system with ultrasonographic registration.

Neurosurgery. 1997;41(3):608–13; discussion 613–604.

15. Ji S, Roberts DW, Hartov A, Paulsen KD. Combining multiple true 3D ultrasound image volumes through re-registration and rasterization. Med Image Comput Comput Assist Interv. 2009;12(Pt 1):795–802.

16. Jodicke A, Deinsberger W, Erbe H, Kriete A, Boker DK. Intraoperative three-dimensional ultrasonography: an approach to register brain shift using multidimensional image processing. Minim Invasive Neurosurg. 1998;41(1):13–9.

17. Keles GE, Lamborn KR, Berger MS. Coregistration accuracy and detection of brain shift using intraoperative sononavigation during resection of hemispheric tumors. Neurosurgery. 2003;53(3):556–64.

18. Koivukangas J, Louhisalmi Y, Alakuijala J, Oikarinen J. Ultrasound-controlled neuronavigator-guided brain surgery. J Neurosurg. 1993;79(1):36–42.

19. Lindner D, Trantakis C, Renner C, Arnold S, Schmitgen A, Schneider J, Meixensberger J. Application of intraoperative 3D ultrasound during navigated tumor resection. Minim Invasive Neurosurg. 2006;49(4):197–202.

20. Lindseth F, Lango T, Bang J, Nagelhus Hernes TA. Accuracy evaluation of a 3D ultrasound-based neuronavigation system. Comput Aided Surg. 2002;7(4):197–222.

21. Lindseth F, Lovstakken L, Rygh OM, Tangen GA, Torp H, Unsgaard G. Blood flow imaging: an angle-independent ultrasound modality for intraoperative assessment of flow dynamics in neurovascular surgery. Neurosurgery. 2009;65(6 Suppl):149–57; discussion 157.

22. Lindseth F, Tangen GA, Lango T, Bang J. Probe calibration for freehand 3-D ultrasound. Ultrasound Med Biol. 2003;29(11):1607–23.

23. Maes F, Collignon A, Vandermeulen D, Marchal G, Suetens P. Multimodality image registration by maximization of mutual information. IEEE Trans Med Imaging. 1997;16(2):187–98.

24. Maes F, Vandermeulen D, Suetens P. Comparative evaluation of multiresolution optimization strategies for multimodality image registration by maximization of mutual information. Med Image Anal. 1999;3(4):373–86.

25. Mathiesen T, Peredo I, Edner G, Kihlstrom L, Svensson M, Ulfarsson E, Andersson T. Neuronavigation for arteriovenous malformation surgery by intraoperative three-dimensional ultrasound angiography. Neurosurgery. 2007;60(4 Suppl 2):345–50; discussion 350–341.

26. Mercier L, Araujo D, Haegelen C, Del Maestro RF, Petrecca K, Collins DL. Registering pre- and postresection 3-dimensional ultrasound for improved visualization of residual brain tumor. Ultrasound Med Biol. 2013;39(1):16–29.

27. Mercier L, Lango T, Lindseth F, Collins DL. A review of calibration techniques for freehand 3-D ultrasound systems. Ultrasound Med Biol. 2005;31(4):449–71.

28. Miller D, Benes L, Sure U. Stand-alone 3D-ultrasound navigation after failure of conventional image guidance for deep-seated lesions. Neurosurg Rev. 2011;34(3):381–7; discussion 387–388.

29. Miller D, Heinze S, Tirakotai W, Bozinov O, Surucu O, Benes L, Bertalanffy H, Sure U. Is the image guidance of ultrasonography beneficial for neurosurgical routine? Surg Neurol. 2007;67(6):579–87; discussion 587–578.

30. Miller D, Lippert C, Vollmer F, Bozinov O, Benes L, Schulte DM, Sure U. Comparison of different reconstruction algorithms for three-dimensional ultrasound imaging in a neurosurgical setting. Int J Med Robot. 2012;8(3):348–59.

31. Moiyadi AV, Shetty PM, Mahajan A, Udare A, Sridhar E. Usefulness of three-dimensional navigable intraoperative ultrasound in resection of brain tumors with a special emphasis on malignant gliomas. Acta Neurochir (Wien). 2013;155(12):2217–25.

32. Muns A, Meixensberger J, Arnold S, Schmitgen A, Arlt F, Chalopin C, Lindner D. Integration of a 3D ultrasound probe into neuronavigation. Acta Neurochir (Wien). 2011;153(7):1529–33.

33. Nabavi A, Black PM, Gering DT, Westin CF, Mehta V, Pergolizzi Jr RS, Ferrant M, Warfield SK, Hata N, Schwartz RB, Wells 3rd WM, Kikinis R, Jolesz FA. Serial intraoperative magnetic resonance imaging of brain shift. Neurosurgery. 2001;48(4):787–97; discussion 797–788.

34. Nagelhus Hernes TA, Lindseth F, Selbekk T, Wollf A, Solberg OV, Harg E, Rygh OM, Tangen GA, Rasmussen I, Augdal S, Couweleers F, Unsgaard G. Computer-assisted 3D ultrasound-guided neurosurgery: technological contributions, including multimodal registration and advanced display, demonstrating future perspectives. Int J Med Robot. 2006;2(1):45–59.

35. Nimsky C, Ganslandt O, Cerny S, Hastreiter P, Greiner G, Fahlbusch R. Quantification of, visualization of, and compensation for brain shift using intraoperative magnetic resonance imaging. Neurosurgery. 2000;47(5):1070–9; discussion 1079–1080.

36. Ohue S, Kumon Y, Nagato S, Kohno S, Harada H, Nakagawa K, Kikuchi K, Miki H, Ohnishi T. Evaluation of intraoperative brain shift using an ultrasound-linked navigation system for brain tumor surgery. Neurol Med Chir (Tokyo). 2010;50(4):291–300.

37. Pagoulatos N, Haynor DR, Kim Y. A fast calibration method for 3-D tracking of ultrasound images using a spatial localizer. Ultrasound Med Biol. 2001;27(9):1219–29.

38. Peredo-Harvey I, Lilja A, Mathiesen T. Postcraniotomy neuronavigation based purely on intraoperative ultrasound imaging without preoperative neuronavigational planning. Neurosurg Rev. 2012;35(2):263–8; discussion 268.

39. Prada F, Del Bene M, Mattei L, Lodigiani L, DeBeni S, Kolev V, Vetrano I, Solbiati L, Sakas G, DiMeco

F. Preoperative magnetic resonance and intraoperative ultrasound fusion imaging for real-time neuronavigation in brain tumor surgery. Ultraschall Med. 2015;36(2):174–86.

40. Rasmussen Jr IA, Lindseth F, Rygh OM, Berntsen EM, Selbekk T, Xu J, Nagelhus Hernes TA, Harg E, Haberg A, Unsgaard G. Functional neuronavigation combined with intra-operative 3D ultrasound: initial experiences during surgical resections close to eloquent brain areas and future directions in automatic brain shift compensation of preoperative data. Acta Neurochir (Wien). 2007;149(4):365–78.

41. Reinertsen I, Lindseth F, Askeland C, Iversen DH, Unsgard G. Intra-operative correction of brain-shift. Acta Neurochir (Wien). 2014;156(7):1301–10.

42. Renovanz M, Hickmann AK, Henkel C, Nadji-Ohl M, Hopf NJ. Navigated versus non-navigated Intraoperative ultrasound: is there any impact on the extent of resection of high-grade gliomas? A retrospective clinical analysis. J Neurol Surg A Cent Eur Neurosurg. 2014;75(3):224–30.

43. Roberts DW, Miga MI, Hartov A, Eisner S, Lemery JM, Kennedy FE, Paulsen KD. Intraoperatively updated neuroimaging using brain modeling and sparse data. Neurosurgery. 1999;45(5):1199–206; discussion 1206–1197.

44. Rygh OM, Nagelhus Hernes TA, Lindseth F, Selbekk T, Brostrup Muller T, Unsgaard G. Intraoperative navigated 3-dimensional ultrasound angiography in tumor surgery. Surg Neurol. 2006;66(6):581–92; discussion 592.

45. Saether CA, Torsteinsen M, Torp SH, Sundstrom S, Unsgard G, Solheim O. Did survival improve after the implementation of intraoperative neuronavigation and 3D ultrasound in glioblastoma surgery? A retrospective analysis of 192 primary operations. J Neurol Surg A Cent Eur Neurosurg. 2012;73(2):73–8.

46. Selbekk T, Jakola AS, Solheim O, Johansen TF, Lindseth F, Reinertsen I, Unsgard G. Ultrasound imaging in neurosurgery: approaches to minimize surgically induced image artefacts for improved resection control. Acta Neurochir (Wien). 2013;155(6):973–80.

47. Solberg OV, Lindseth F, Bo LE, Muller S, Bakeng JB, Tangen GA, Hernes TA. 3D ultrasound reconstruction algorithms from analog and digital data. Ultrasonics. 2011;51(4):405–19.

48. Solberg OV, Lindseth F, Torp H, Blake RE, Nagelhus Hernes TA. Freehand 3D ultrasound reconstruction algorithms--a review. Ultrasound Med Biol. 2007;33(7):991–1009.

49. Sure U, Benes L, Bozinov O, Woydt M, Tirakotai W, Bertalanffy H. Intraoperative landmarking of vascular anatomy by integration of duplex and Doppler ultra-sonography in image-guided surgery. Technical note. Surg Neurol. 2005;63(2):133–41; discussion 141–132.

50. Tirakotai W, Miller D, Heinze S, Benes L, Bertalanffy H, Sure U. A novel platform for image-guided ultrasound. Neurosurgery. 2006;58(4):710–8; discussion 710–718.

51. Trantakis C, Meixensberger J, Lindner D, Strauss G, Grunst G, Schmidtgen A, Arnold S. Iterative neuronavigation using 3D ultrasound. A feasibility study. Neurol Res. 2002;24(7):666–70.

52. Trobaugh JW, Richard WD, Smith KR, Bucholz RD. Frameless stereotactic ultrasonography: method and applications. Comput Med Imaging Graph. 1994;18(4):235–46.

53. Unsgaard G, Ommedal S, Rygh OM, Lindseth F. Operation of arteriovenous malformations assisted by stereoscopic navigation-controlled display of preoperative magnetic resonance angiography and intraoperative ultrasound angiography. Neurosurgery. 2005;56 Suppl 2:281–90.

54. Unsgaard G, Rygh OM, Selbekk T, Muller TB, Kolstad F, Lindseth F, Hernes TA. Intra-operative 3D ultrasound in neurosurgery. Acta Neurochir (Wien). 2006;148(3):235–53; discussion 253.

55. Unsgaard G, Selbekk T, Brostrup Muller T, Ommedal S, Torp SH, Myhr G, Bang J, Nagelhus Hernes TA. Ability of navigated 3D ultrasound to delineate gliomas and metastases – comparison of image interpretations with histopathology. Acta Neurochir (Wien). 2005;147(12):1259–69; discussion 1269.

56. Unsgaard G, Solheim O, Lindseth F, Selbekk T. Intraoperative imaging with 3D ultrasound in neurosurgery. Acta Neurochir Suppl. 2011;109:181–6.

57. Wells 3rd WM, Viola P, Atsumi H, Nakajima S, Kikinis R. Multi-modal volume registration by maximization of mutual information. Med Image Anal. 1996;1(1):35–51.

58. Willems PW, Taphoorn MJ, Burger H, Berkelbach van der Sprenkel JW, Tulleken CA. Effectiveness of neuronavigation in resecting solitary intracerebral contrast-enhancing tumors: a randomized controlled trial. J Neurosurg. 2006;104(3):360–8.

59. Wirtz CR, Albert FK, Schwaderer M, Heuer C, Staubert A, Tronnier VM, Knauth M, Kunze S. The benefit of neuronavigation for neurosurgery analyzed by its impact on glioblastoma surgery. Neurol Res. 2000;22(4):354–60.

60. Zhou H, Miller D, Schulte DM, Benes L, Rosenow F, Bertalanffy H, Sure U. Transsulcal approach supported by navigation-guided neurophysiological monitoring for resection of paracentral cavernomas. Clin Neurol Neurosurg. 2009;111(1):69–78.

Part V

Contrast Enhanced Ultrasound (CEUS)

Contrast-Enhanced Ultrasound: Basic Principles, General Application, and Future Trends

12

Marcello Caremani, Carla Richetta, and Daniela Caremani

12.1 Contrast-Enhanced Ultrasound (CEUS)

Ultrasound (US) is a real-time, low-cost, noninvasive, and widely available imaging tool which is nowadays well established in clinical routine. B-mode images can provide good discrimination between pathologic and healthy tissue and, with the introduction of Doppler images, it is feasible to achieve good visualization of vessels and to measure blood flow direction and speed thus widening the diagnostic range. Nevertheless, sometimes signal detection is unsatisfactory for diagnostic purposes since it cannot be easily distinguished from background noise. This is typical for masses sited in very deep regions of the abdomen. Furthermore, both B-mode and Doppler have the drawback of being unable to highlight microvasculature, and Doppler cannot detect low flow systems such as capillaries. Doppler techniques show also some other disadvantages such as the impossibility to study more than one or few vessels at a time and signal changes when modifying the insonation angle. Because of all these reasons, research focused on developing agents able to amplify signals coming from the region of interest, i.e., pathological masses, called ultrasound contrast agents. US contrast media are able to modify acoustic impedance of tissues while interacting with incident beam and thus increasing ecogenicity and blood backscattering [1]: US contrast media in fact, when insonated by an ultrasound beam, undergo a series of contractions and expansions with a frequency depending from their dimensions, thus acting like an ultrasound source themselves with radial ultrasounds emission.

Ideal US contrast agent characteristics are high ecogenicity, linear relationship between concentration and signal intensity, ability to cross the pulmonary capillary bed, stability over the duration of the procedure, minimal imaging artifacts, and low toxicity [2]. Furthermore, US contrast agents, compared to gadolinium and iodinate contrast agents, are called "blood pool", since they remain inside the vascular tree instead of

M. Caremani, MD (✉)
Radiology Unit, Department of Infectious Diseases, Ospedale S. Donatovia P. Nenni 20, Arezzo 52100, Italy
e-mail: m.caremani@gmail.com

C. Richetta
Department of Neurosurgery, Fondazione IRCCS Istituto Neurologico C. Besta, Milan, Italy

D. Caremani
Department of Infectious Diseases, Section of Anatomical Pathology, Ospedale S. Donato, via P. Nenni 20, Arezzo 52100, Italy

spreading in the interstitial space. This characteristic makes them so powerful in highlighting both macro- and microvasculature and explains why only arterial phase is similar between all these imaging modalities [1–3].

Back to the 1960s, cardiologists started to wonder if right-left cardiac shunt could be evaluated with the intravenous injection of substances acting as contrast agents, detecting them inside the left cardiac chambers. At that time, transpulmonary contrast agents able to cross the pulmonary filter and reach the systemic circulation were still not available. The first applications of transpulmonary agents (3–5 µ diameter) date back to the 1990s, and they were combined with echo-color Doppler (ECD) to improve echocardiography, transcranial Doppler (TCD), and evaluation of portal vein and renal arteries. The main limitations were Doppler artifacts and the impossibility to study the capillary bed with Doppler techniques even after contrast media usage [4]. These contrast agents, called first-generation contrast agents, were microbubbles containing air surrounded by a thin lipidic, proteic, or polymeric shell. The first contrast medium introduced in the clinical routine was Levovist® which had a shell composed of galactose and palmitic acid. Because of their air core, first-generation microbubbles are unstable: they may be destroyed already during the preparation and injection or while flowing through the capillary bed. Hence, they can be visualized only for a limited number of acquisitions. Moreover, if injected in bolus, they constantly produce a sovra-amplification artifact called blooming, which makes the signal to appear also outside the vessels. This side effect can be avoided by injecting microbubbles slowly with a continuous infusion, but this makes dynamic studies not feasible [5, 6].

In the last decade, microbubbles containing injectable gases with a lower diffusion coefficient were developed such as SonoVue®. Research also focused on their shell adding phospholipids, thus creating more elastic and stable microbubbles [7]. SonoVue ® contains sulfur hexafluoride which is eliminated through respiration, while the shell undergo hepatic metabolization without involving kidneys like gadolinium or iodinate agents.

Essentially a 2–4 ml contrast medium bolus is manually injected in a peripheral vein through a 18–20 G pipe. After intravenous injection, the contrast agent last up to 5 min, before being completely disrupted. Generally, US contrast media are very well tolerated with an incidence of adverse events around 0.009 % being the most safe drugs in medicine [8, 9]. However, since allergic and idiosyncratic effects have been described in the past, the exam should be performed in a protected environment where resuscitation can be feasible [10]. Nor steroids or antihistamine drugs have been proven effective for prophylaxis. Also mild reactions such as migraine, vertigo, erythema, and pain in the injection area have been described with an incidence of 2 %. However, it is recommended to keep the patient under observation for at least 30 min after the end of the exam even if usually adverse events tend to show within the first 3 min. Contrast media are not allowed in pregnant women and children; restrictions during breastfeeding are effective only in some countries. The main microbubble contraindications were defined in 2007 by EMEA, and they include: previous or ongoing myocardial infarction, known left-right cardiac shunt, severe pulmonary hypertension, noncontrolled arterial hypertension, adult distress respiratory syndrome, severe arrhythmias, and stage IV heart failure. Because of this, patients need to sign an informed consent before undergoing the procedure.

Second-generation microbubbles show also the capability to resonate even if stimulated with low-intensity ultrasound while, in this condition, first-generation microbubbles remain inert. Depending on incident ultrasound beam power and on the pressure they are subjected to, contrast agents show different behaviors. Generally, we distinguish between high-mechanical index and low-mechanical index techniques. Mechanical index is the result of the ratio between the peak of acoustic negative pressure (measured in MPa) and the square root of the central frequency of the frequency band in use (measured in MHz) [11]. With high MI techniques (>1 MPa), it is possible to obtain a transitory echo signal from contrast media due to microbubble destruction and leading to an "intermittent imaging." Low MI techniques (<100 KPa) can be used only with second-generation microbubbles to achieve a continuous real-time image acquisition. These techniques are based on nondestructive microbubble oscillation hence without disruption and consequent consumption of contrast agents, thanks to the coincidence between US frequencies and second-generation microbubbles intrinsic resonance frequency. Microbubble oscillation is nonlinear because the diameter in expansion is superior than the contraction scattering ultrasound with a frequency different from the incident (fundamental) one and are called harmonic frequencies. These include subharmonics, ultraharmonics, and multiple of the fundamental frequency. At present, 2nd harmonic is used to produce the images obtained from microbubble oscillation, since the subsequent harmonics are of decreasing amplitude and thus inadequate to generate a proper signal [12]. Selectively filtering out the fundamental frequency allows transducer to receive only the harmonic frequency. Main advantages of harmonic imaging over conventional US are increased axial and lateral resolution, decreased reverberation and side-lobe artifacts, and increased signal-to-noise ratio.

Beside cardiology, CEUS is a well-established methodology especially in hepatology where it was proven to be superior to B-mode and basically is now considered to be at the same level of computed tomography (CT) and magnetic resonance imaging (MRI) in highlighting liver lesion features, and its usage is properly coded by international guidelines. For example, CEUS is able to underline contrastographic behavior of hepatocarcinoma characterized by typical arterial phase enhancement followed by a washout phase along the portal phase (Figs. 12.1 and 12.2).

It is also a very sensitive method to detect and typify secondary lesions, both hyper- and hypovascular, which cannot be visualized with conventional US (Fig. 12.3). There is a strong indication for hepatic angioma diagnosis as well and focal nodular hyperplasia, while CEUS use along and after ablation therapy is still a matter of discussion. Other extrahepatic applications include biliary tract, lungs and lymphnodes visu-

alization, differential diagnosis between pancreatic neoformations such as adenocarcinoma and neuroendocrine tumors, differentiation between splenic infarct and splenic lymphomatous lesions [13], abdominal trauma assessment [14]. Another application is the study of vascular endoprosthesis especially when leaking is suspected and, recently, the detection and characterization of brain lesions during the surgical excision.

Lesion characterization with CEUS is mainly qualitative or semiquantitative and thus dependent on the operator's skills and experience and hardly reproducible. To increase objectivity of the obtained results, specific softwares allowing quantitative evaluation, especially regarding perfusion, have been recently developed. Mostly all these softwares are able to analyze DICOM data which are the ordinary format of PACS. After processing data, the software allows to obtain multiple parametric images representing selected areas in different colors according to a colorimetric scale coding differences in perfusion (necrotic areas appear blue and wider in high-grade lesions, while low-grade neoplasms are more homogeneous), an Excel file containing perfusion parameters values, and a time-intensity curve (TIC) for each region of interest (ROI) selected. The quantitative parameters usually calculated are (Fig. 12.4):

Peak of enhancement (PE): it is the maximum intensity measured in the TIC curve.
Raising time (RT): it expresses the time from the instant at which the maximum slope tangent intersects the x-axis to the peak of the fitted curve.
Mean transit time (mTTI): it is the expression of the time a certain volume of blood spent in the capillary circulation inside the ROI.
Time to peak (TTP): it expresses the time from time origin to the peak of the fitted curve.
Wash in time (Wi): it is the time from 5 to 95 % of intensity.
Washout time (Wo): it is the time from the peak to the lowest intensity.
Area under curve (AUC): it is the area under the TIC curve above the baseline calculated from time zero (t_0) to the end of washout.

Fig. 12.1 Wide echogenic lesion of VII hepatic segment in a cirrhotic liver showing enhancement after UCSs administration

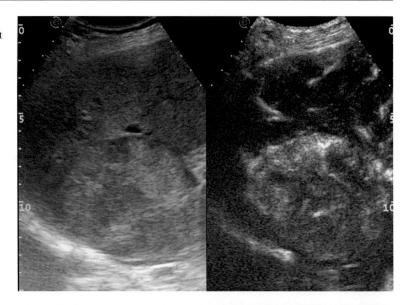

Fig. 12.2 Hepatocarcinoma. Late washout and tendency to hyperechogenicity

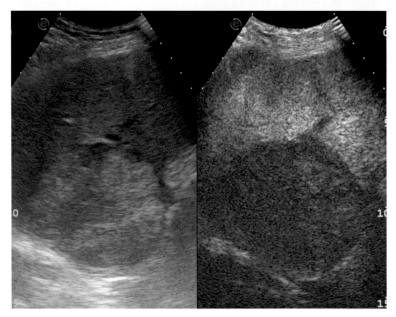

Falling time (FT): it is the equivalent of RT on the descending side of the curve.

Quality of fitting (QOF): this parameter tells us how reliable and representative of the reality the linearized data are. TIC with a QOF less than 70 % should be discarded.

In some fields, a solid expertise in CEUS and perfusion quantification techniques is already a fact. Perfusion quantification with specific off-line software shows advantages in order to identify specific pathological situations such as acute rejection after kidney transplant or gastrointestinal inflammatory diseases [15, 16]. Moreover, quantification of some parameters such us time to peak (TTP), mean transit time (mTTI) in the capillaries, regional blood flow, and regional blood volume in breast cancer shows good correlation with MRI images [17]. Interestingly, morphologic analysis of the curve allowed to

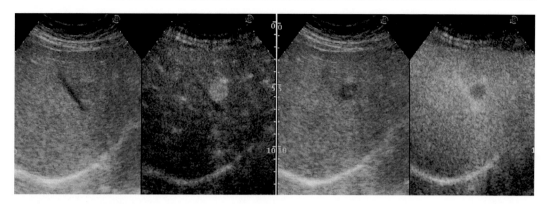

Fig. 12.3 Hepatic metastatic lesion. Tumor is isoechogenic to parenchyma showing intense enhancement after UCS administration. And then a rapid washout, hypoechogenicity along the portal phase

Fig. 12.4 Typical TIC after intravenous bolus injection of microbubbles. The software converts video data (pixel intensity) into echo-power data (arbitrary units (a.u.)) which are directly proportional to the instantaneous concentration of microbubbles in the area of interest. This process is called linearization

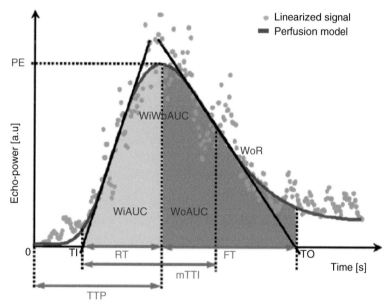

detect different patterns strongly related to the histology of the mammary lesion. Since CEUS has the potential to highlight the capillary circulation, it can be useful in the evaluation of cutaneous flaps perfusion in order to predict future complications [18]. Another promising application of this new technique is represented by its use in the follow-up of patients in treatment with antiangiogenetic drugs. This may allow to differentiate between patient responders and nonresponders [19, 20]. Especially the parameter area under curve (AUC) after 1 month of treatment seems to be a good predictor of the outcome after 6 months in gastrointestinal stromal tumors

(GIST), renal cells tumors, and hepatocellular carcinoma.

Recently perfusion quantification has been explored in the neurosurgical field along brain tumor surgical excision (Figs. 12.5 and 12.6).

Even though CEUS shows many strength points, with the development of molecular imaging techniques and the growing demand for a more personalized and hyper-specialized medicine, a single imaging modality appears no longer satisfactory [21]. It is a matter of fact that each imaging model carries its own limitations and key strengths. For example, MRI is a soft-tissue contrast imaging modality with high spatial

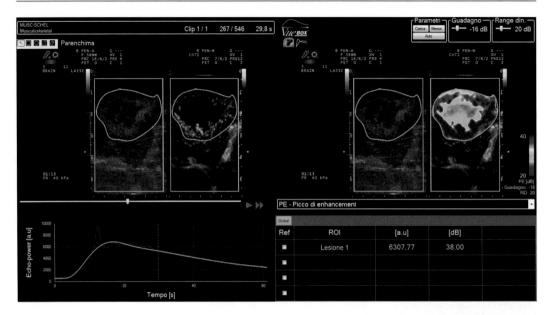

Fig. 12.5 Frontal panel obtained at the end of the analysis of a brain lesion. The selected green area represents the lesion (GBM). On the top, original and parametric images are displayed. On the bottom, the time-intensity curve is shown together with quantitative parameters table reporting PE in the present case

resolution and multi-planar imaging capacities, but its cost is relatively high and it is not a real-time modality while US is a real-time, low-cost, nonionizing, and widely available imaging tool, but its resolution is low and largely depends on the analysis of operator. On the other hand, fluorescence imaging is an imaging technique with high sensitivity and multicolor, but it is non-quantitative with poor tissue penetrating ability [22]. Because of this over the past few years, the possibility to integrate different imaging modalities gained great interest in healthcare industry in order to merge together the most relevant properties of each modality, hence obtaining the highest readout and increasing clinical efficacy [23]. The complementary use of the two nonionizing modalities US and MRI is of great interest. MRI-US fusion is a product of the last decade which already gave promising results in brain surgery [24, 25] (Fig. 12.7), urology guiding prostate biopsy [26], prenatal diagnosis [27], and targeting of liver tumors amenable for thermal ablation [28].

To increase the sensitivity and specificity of modalities fusion, an injectable micro-/nano-device supporting multimodality imaging could

be of great value [29]. Microbubbles functionalized with different ligands can work in this way, and so they have been investigated worldwide as a potential multimodal contrast agent [23]. Both lipidic and polymeric microbubbles may be loaded with different particles and drugs, but the latter show additional potentialities. They are more robust; thus, they have a longer half-life, they possess greatly improved drug-loading capabilities, and they are easily synthesized in a one-pot reaction [30].

The functionalization of microbubbles with supermagnetic iron oxide nanoparticles (SPIONs) or radioactive tracers makes them visible through MRI [29–31] and CT/SPECT [23], respectively, enabling visualization of many information, both functional and anatomical, and improving diagnostic possibilities. Moreover, microbubbles can be stabilized by embedded magnetic nanoparticles into the bubble shell, and they can be guided by magnetic fields to the region of interest [31, 32]. Some studies conducted on animals showed that biodistribution between different organs may be modified using different ligands [23]. This should be taken into account in patients with specific diseases and thus when unable to properly

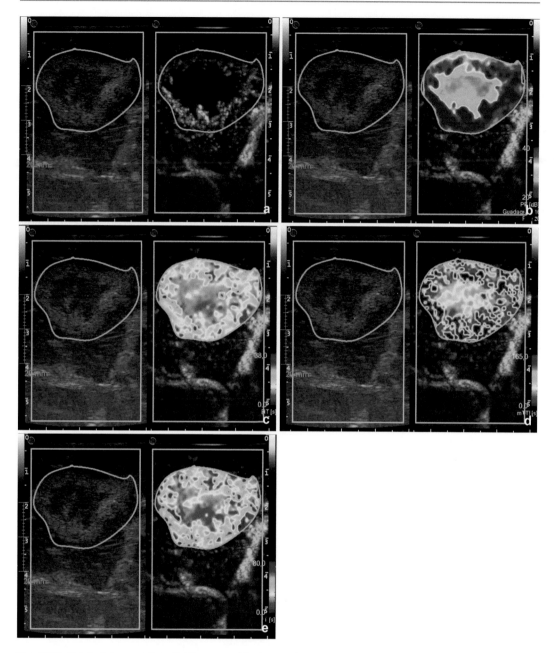

Fig. 12.6 Original image of a glioblastoma with the selected region of interest (ROI) (**a**); parametric images representing some of the calculated parameters: peak of enhancement (PE) (**b**), raising time (RT) (**c**), mean transit time (mTTI) (**d**), falling time (FT) (**e**)

clear the organism from the contrast agent. Furthermore, functionalization with ligands able to bind molecules expressed in specific diseases allows a highly specific in vivo noninvasive molecular imaging. Since microbubbles display a intravascular nature, they can bind to altered phe-notypes of cells present in the intravascular compartment [33]. This limits a number of targets which are expressed in the extravascular tissue. The bond between the ligand and the target should be specific, rapid, and strong since shear forces may disrupt it by moving the bubbles away

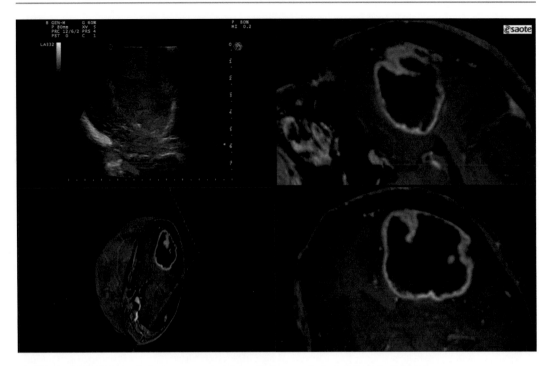

Fig. 12.7 US-MRI fusion in brain surgery during surgical removal of a left frontal glioblastoma

from the target in a very short time. Ideally the ligand should not have any pharmacological effects in order to avoid any increase of adverse effects [33]. Because of this, antibodies are clinically less desirable since they can lead to immunological reactions linked to manufacturing issues [34]. Nevertheless antibodies are useful in validation and proof-of-concept studies since they have a high specificity towards the target [33]. Other kinds of ligands, such as small peptides, aptamers, and lectins, show the advantage of being easier to manipulate compared to antibodies, for example, they can be directly incorporated in the microbubble shell instead of being conjugated using the biotin-streptavidin linker [35, 36].

Different binding ligands have been explored for targeting intravascular molecules such as integrins and, specifically, the triplet Arg-Gli-Asp (RGD). These integrins, together with vascular endothelial growth factor type 2 (VEGFR2), are highly expressed in vessels activated by inflammation and tumor angiogenesis [37]. Overexpression of VEGFR2 and/or VEGF has been associated with progression and unfavor-

able prognosis in many tumors such as colorectal, gastric, and pancreatic carcinoma but also in breast and prostate carcinoma and in malignant glioma and melanoma [37]. Therefore, molecular ultrasound can be a useful tool in oncology applications for the detection of integrin and VEGF/VEGFR2 expression in suspected tissue and assessment of changes during diseases progression or after peculiar treatments such as anti-angiogenetic drugs [38–40]. Some preclinical studies have already been carried out with integrin/VEGFR2-targeted microbubbles invariably showing a correlation between targeted bubble retention by tissues and integrin expression [39–44].

In addition to their diagnostic properties, microbubbles have a potentiality for therapeutic purposes. Through US excitation, bubbles undergo repetitive contractions and expansions inducing microstreaming around the microbubbles that lead to channel modulation, thus affecting cells permeability [45]. Stronger US pressure may even induce bubbles disruption producing a shock wave that can cause a perforation through the cell membrane and blood vessel permeabilization [46, 47]. This mechanical properties can be of great value in the delivery of chemotherapeutic agents loaded in the bubble shell especially through high selective membranes, for instance, the blood-brain barrier (BBB) [48, 49].

References

1. Catalano A, Farina R (2012) Mezzi di Contrasto in Ecografia CEUS. Metodologia di impiego e Indicazioni cliniche. E.L.I. Medica, Villaricca, Italy
2. Correas JM, Bridal L, Lesavre A, Méjean A, Claudon M, Hélénon O (2001) Ultrasound contrast agents: properties, principles of action, tolerance, and artifacts. Eur Radiol 11(8):1316–1328
3. Catalano O, Siani A (2007) Ecografia in Oncologia. Testo-atlante di Ultrasonografia diagnostica interventistica nei tumori. I edizione. Spinger, Pagg 36–57
4. Bertolotto M, Catalano O (2009) Contrast-enhanced ultrasound: past, present, and future. Ultrasound Clin 4(3):339–367. doi:10.1016/j.cult.2009.10.011
5. Forsberger F et al (1994) Artifacts in ultrasonic contrast agent studies. J Ultrasound Med 13:357–365
6. Goldberg BB (ed) (1997) Ultrasound contrast agents. Martin Dunitz, London
7. Leong-Poi H, Song J, Rim S-J, Christiansen J, Kaul S, Lindner JR (2002) Influence of microbubble shell properties on ultrasound signal: implications for low-power perfusion imaging. J Am Soc Echocardiogr 15(10 Pt 2):1269–1276
8. Ter Haar G (2008) Bubble trouble? Ultraschall Med 29(5):550–551. doi:10.1055/s-0028-1098033
9. Torzilli G (2005) Adverse effects associated with SonoVue use. Expert Opin Drug Saf 4(3):399–401. doi:10.1517/14740338.4.3.399
10. Van Camp G, Droogmans S, Cosyns B (2007) Bio-effects of ultrasound contrast agents in daily clinical practice: fact or fiction? Eur Heart J 28(10):1190–1192
11. Humphrey VF (2007) Ultrasound and matter – physical interactions. Prog Biophys Mol Biol 93(1–3):195–211. doi:10.1016/j.pbiomolbio.2006.07.024
12. Choudhry S, Gorman B, Charboneau JW, Tradup DJ, Beck RJ, Kofler JM, Groth DS (2000) Comparison of tissue harmonic imaging with conventional US in abdominal disease. Radiographics 20(4):1127–1135. doi:10.1148/radiographics.20.4.g00jl371127
13. Piscaglia F, Nolsoe C, Dietrich CF et al (2012) The EFSUMB guidelines and recommendations on the clinical practice of contrast enhanced ultrasound (CEUS): update 2011 on non-hepatic applications. Ultraschall Med 33(1):33–59
14. Catalano O, Aiani A, Barozzi L et al (2009) CEUS in abdominal trauma: multi-center study. Abdom Imaging 34:225–234
15. Correas J-M, Claudon M, Tranquart F, Hélénon AO (2006) The kidney: imaging with microbubble contrast agents. Ultrasound Q 22(1):53–66
16. Girlich C, Jung EM, Huber E, Ott C, Iesalnieks I, Schreyer A, Schacherer D (2011) Comparison between preoperative quantitative assessment of bowel wall vascularization by contrast-enhanced ultrasound and operative macroscopic findings and results of histopathological scoring in Crohn's disease. Ultraschall Med (Stuttgart, Germany: 1980) 32(2):154–159. doi:10.1055/s-0029-1245398
17. Caproni N, Marchisio F, Pecchi A, Canossi B, Battista R, D'Alimonte P, Torricelli P (2010) Contrast-enhanced ultrasound in the characterisation of breast masses: utility of quantitative analysis in comparison with MRI. Eur Radiol 20(6):1384–1395. doi:10.1007/s00330-009-1690-1
18. Geis S, Prantl L, Gehmert S, Lamby P, Nerlich M, Angele P, Jung EM (2011) TTP (time to PEAK) and RBV (regional blood volume) as valuable parameters to detect early flap failure. Clin Hemorheol Microcirc 48(1):81–94. doi:10.3233/CH-2011-1396
19. Cosgrove D, Lassau N (2010) Imaging of perfusion using ultrasound. Eur J Nucl Med Mol Imaging 37(Suppl 1):S65–S85. doi:10.1007/s00259-010-1537-7
20. Lassau N, Chami L, Chebil M, Benatsou B, Bidault S, Girard E, Roche A (2011) Dynamic contrast-enhanced ultrasonography (DCE-US) and anti-angiogenic treatments. Discov Med 11(56):18–24
21. Lin Y, Chen Z-Y, Yang F (2013) Ultrasound-based multimodal molecular imaging and functional ultrasound contrast agents. Curr Pharm Des 19(18):3342–3351
22. Cheng X, Li H, Chen Y, Luo B, Liu X, Liu W, Haibo X, Yang X (2013) Ultrasound-triggered phase transition sensitive magnetic fluorescent nanodroplets as a multimodal imaging contrast agent in rat and mouse model. PlosOne. doi:10.1371/journal.pone.0085003
23. Barrefelt AA et al (2013) Multimodality imaging using SPECT/CT and MRI and ligand functionalized 99mTc-labeled magnetic microbubbles. EJNMMI Res 3:12. doi:10.1186/2191-219X-3-12
24. Schlaier JR, Warnat J, Dorenbeck U, Proescholdt M, Schebesch K-M, Brawanski A (2004) Image fusion of MR images and real-time ultrasonography: evaluation of fusion accuracy combining two commercial instruments, a neuronavigation system and a ultrasound system. Acta Neurochir 146(3):271–276. doi:10.1007/s00701-003-0155-6; discussion 276–277
25. Prada F, Del Bene M, Mattei L, Lodigiani L, DeBeni S, Kolev V, DiMeco F (2015) Preoperative magnetic resonance and intraoperative ultrasound fusion imaging for real-time neuronavigation in brain tumor surgery. Ultraschall Med (Stuttgart, Germany: 1980) 36(2):174–186. doi:10.1055/s-0034-1385347
26. Marks L, Young S, Natarajan S (2013) MRI-ultrasound fusion for guidance of targeted prostate biopsy. Curr Opin Urol 23(1):43–50. doi:10.1097/MOU.0b013e32835ad3ee
27. Salomon LJ, Bernard J-P, Millischer A-E, Sonigo P, Brunelle F, Boddaert N, Ville Y (2013) MRI and ultrasound fusion imaging for prenatal diagnosis. Am J Obstet Gynecol 209(2):148.e1–9. doi:10.1016/j.ajog.2013.05.031

28. Mauri G, Cova L, De Beni S, Ierace T, Tondolo T, Cerri A, Goldberg SN, Solbiati L (2015) Real-time US-CT/MRI image fusion for guidance of thermal ablation of liver tumors undetectable with US: results in 295 cases. Cardiovasc Intervent Radiol 38(1):143–151. doi:10.1007/s00270-014-0897-y

29. Brismar TB, Grishenkov D, Gustafsson B, Härmark J, Barrefelt A, Kothapalli SV, Margheritelli S, Oddo L, Caidahl K, Hebert H, Paradossi G (2012) Magnetite nanoparticles can be coupled to microbubbles to support multimodal imaging. Biomacromolecules 13(5):1390–1399. doi:10.1021/bm300099f

30. Nakatsuka MA, Lee JH, Nakayama E, Hung AM, Hsu MJ, Mattrey RF, Goodwin AP (2011) Facile one-pot synthesis of polymer-phospholipid composite microbubbles with enhanced drug loading capacity for ultrasound-triggered therapy. Soft Matt 2011(7):1656–1659. doi:10.1039/C0SM01131B

31. Cai X, Yang F, Ning G (2012) Applications of magnetic microbubbles for theranostics. Theranostics 2(1):103–112. doi:10.7150/thno.3464

32. Yang F, Li Y, Chen Z et al (2009) Superparamagnetic iron oxide nanoparticle-embedded encapsulated microbubbles as dual contrast agents of magnetic resonance and ultrasound imaging. Biomaterials 30:3882–3890

33. Moestue SA, Gribbestad IS, Hansen R (2012) Intravascular targets for molecular contrast-enhanced ultrasound imaging. Int J Mol Sci 13(6):6679–6697. doi:10.3390/ijms13066679

34. Jain M, Kamal N, Batra SK (2007) Engineering antibodies for clinical applications. Trends Biotechnol 25(7):307–316. doi:10.1016/j.tibtech.2007.05.001

35. Pillai R, Marinelli ER, Fan H, Nanjappan P, Song B, von Wronski MA, Swenson RE (2010) A phospholipid-PEG2000 conjugate of a vascular endothelial growth factor receptor 2 (VEGFR2)-targeting heterodimer peptide for contrast-enhanced ultrasound imaging of angiogenesis. Bioconjug Chem 21(3):556–562. doi:10.1021/bc9005688

36. Pochon S, Tardy I, Bussat P, Bettinger T, Brochot J, von Wronski M, Schneider M (2010) BR55: a lipopeptide-based VEGFR2-targeted ultrasound contrast agent for molecular imaging of angiogenesis. Invest Radiol 45(2):89–95. doi:10.1097/RLI.0b013e3181c5927c

37. Hicklin DJ, Ellis LM (2005) Role of the vascular endothelial growth factor pathway in tumor growth and angiogenesis. J Clin Oncol 23:1011–1027

38. Kiessling F, Gaetjens J, Palmowski M (2011) Application of molecular ultrasound for imaging integrin expression. Theranostics 1:127–134

39. Korpanty G, Carbon JG, Grayburn PA, Fleming JB, Brekken RA (2007) Monitoring response to anticancer therapy by targeting microbubbles to tumor vasculature. Clin Cancer Res 13(1):323–330. doi:10.1158/1078-0432.CCR-06-1313

40. Palmowski M, Huppert J, Ladewig G, Hauff P, Reinhardt M, Mueller MM, Kiessling F (2008) Molecular profiling of angiogenesis with targeted ultrasound imaging: early assessment of antiangiogenic therapy effects. Mol Cancer Ther 7(1):101–109. doi:10.1158/1535-7163.MCT-07-0409

41. Pysz MA, Foygel K, Rosenberg J, Gambhir SS, Schneider M, Willmann JK (2010) Antiangiogenic cancer therapy: monitoring with molecular US and a clinically translatable contrast agent (BR55). Radiology 256(2):519–527. doi:10.1148/radiol.10091858

42. Willmann JK, Paulmurugan R, Chen K, Gheysens O, Rodriguez-Porcel M, Lutz AM, Gambhir SS (2008) US imaging of tumor angiogenesis with microbubbles targeted to vascular endothelial growth factor receptor type 2 in mice. Radiology 246(2):508–518. doi:10.1148/radiol.2462070536

43. Lee DJ, Lyshchik A, Huamani J, Hallahan DE, Fleischer AC (2008) Relationship between retention of a vascular endothelial growth factor receptor 2 (VEGFR2)-targeted ultrasonographic contrast agent and the level of VEGFR2 expression in an in vivo breast cancer model. J Ultrasound Med 27(6):855–866, Retrieved from http://www.ncbi.nlm.nih.gov/pubmed/18499845

44. Liu H, Chen Y, Yan F, Han X, Wu J, Liu X, Zheng H (2015) Ultrasound molecular imaging of vascular endothelial growth factor receptor 2 expression for endometrial receptivity evaluation. Theranostics 5(2):206–217. doi:10.7150/thno.9847

45. Sboros V (2008) Response of contrast agents to ultrasound. Adv Drug Deliv Rev 60(10):1117–1136. doi:10.1016/j.addr.2008.03.011

46. Mitragotri S (2005) Healing sound: the use of ultrasound in drug delivery and other therapeutic applications. Nat Rev Drug Discov 4(3):255–260. doi:10.1038/nrd1662

47. Dalecki D (2004) Mechanical bioeffects of ultrasound. Annu Rev Biomed Eng 6:229–248. doi:10.1146/annurev.bioeng.6.040803.140126

48. Fan C-H, Lin W-H, Ting C-Y, Chai W-Y, Yen T-C, Liu H-L, Yeh C-K (2014) Contrast-enhanced ultrasound imaging for the detection of focused ultrasound-induced blood–brain barrier opening. Theranostics 4(10):1014–1025. doi:10.7150/thno.9575

49. Liu H-L, Fan C-H, Ting C-Y, Yeh C-K (2014) Combining microbubbles and ultrasound for drug delivery to brain tumors: current progress and overview. Theranostics 4(4):432–444. doi:10.7150/thno.8074

Contrast-Enhanced Ultrasound (CEUS) in Neurosurgery

13

Francesco Prada, Massimiliano Del Bene, and Francesco DiMeco

13.1 Introduction

Contrast agents (CAs) in medical imaging are used to highlight different characteristics of various organs, vessels, and cavities, making their visualization more simple and efficient.

Ultrasound contrast agents (UCAs) had been in use since the 1970s. The first studies regarding first-generation contrast agents were published in the late 1990s. Then second-generation UCAs were released, allowing for a real-time continuous imaging, thanks to low-mechanical index US and contrast-specific algorithm.

Contrast-enhanced ultrasound (CEUS) consists in the real-time continuous visualization of the behavior of UCAs in the tissue of interest. UCAs are suspension of microbubbles (MBs) of gas encoated by a polymeric shell (diameter: 2–6 μm) that behave as purely intravascular contrast agents [1–3].

The pharmacokinetics of the MBs is quite different from that of CAs used for CT and MRI which generally diffuse in the interstitial space [4]. CEUS has a number of distinct advantages over CT and MRI. It can be performed immediately, without any preliminary laboratory testing, and it can be carried out in different settings such as outpatient's clinic or surgical theatre. Furthermore, it allows a true real-time continuous imaging and has the potential to depict rapid changes.

Second-generation US contrast agents are clinically safe and well tolerated, although many applications continue to be off-label. UCAs registered in Europe are licensed only for cardiac, liver, breast, and vascular applications [1, 5, 6].

CEUS is nowadays an established technique for many organs, as it allows, among other things, better depiction of neoplastic lesions and vascular tree [1, 6].

The main clinically recognized application is the characterization of focal liver lesions: CEUS allows real-time assessment of contrast enhancement and vascularity of focal lesions during the different dynamic phases, after injection of an intravenous contrast agent [6].

There has been exponentially increasing interest in the clinical applications of CEUS, and new fields have been investigated, so that nearly all organ systems have now been subjected to some kind of CEUS study; however, many applications continue to be off-label [1, 5, 6].

A previous version of this chapter represented incorrect order of the authors.

For this reason an erratum has been published, correcting the mistake in the previous version and showing the correct order of the authors (see DOI 10.1007/978-3-319-25268-1_15)

F. Prada • M. Del Bene, MD (✉)
Department of Neurosurgery, Fondazione IRCCS
Istituto Neurologico C. Besta,
via Celoria 11, Milan 20133, Italy
e-mail: macs.delbene@gmail.com

F. DiMeco
Department of Neurosurgery, Fondazione IRCCS
Istituto Neurologico C. Besta,
via Celoria 11, Milan 20133, Italy

Department of Neurosurgery,
Johns Hopkins Medical School, Baltimore, MD, USA

© Springer International Publishing Switzerland 2016
F. Prada et al. (eds.), *Intraoperative Ultrasound (IOUS) in Neurosurgery: From Standard B-mode to Elastosonography*, DOI 10.1007/978-3-319-25268-1_13

It is therefore worthwhile to explore and standardize its application in various fields of neurosurgery, ranging from neuro-oncology and skull-base surgery to vascular surgery, integrating these information to the anatomical and functional ones obtained with standard B-mode and Doppler imaging [2, 3, 7, 8].

To achieve a proper examination, a dedicated equipment is necessary, along with a specific training, in order to standardize the procedure [9].

The examination with CEUS during neurosurgical procedures should be performed following as much as possible the criteria already established for other organs.

Main parameters to be taken into account are timing (arterial and venous phase [time is given as range]), degree of CE (comparison with brain parenchyma), and contrast distribution (centripetal/centrifugal pattern, visibility of afferent/efferent vessels, intralesional vessels, cystic/necrotic areas) [1, 3, 6].

13.2 Exam Technique

13.2.1 US Equipment

CEUS requires a US system with specific algorithm capable to analyze the echo signal in order to represent only the harmonic signal from the UCA and suppressing the linear signal originated from the tissue. The most used probe is the multifrequency (3–11 Mhz) linear array that permits to study both depth and superficial lesions [2, 3, 7, 8]. As UCA, the most used is sulfur hexafluoride (SonoVue™ –Bracco, Italy): a second-generation contrast agent that permits to acquire nonlinear signal at low power of insonation [5]. This feature leads to minimal MB disruption and allows a continuous study of structure/organ for some minutes, dynamically assessing the enhancement in real time.

13.2.2 Operative Setting

Prior to perform whatever intraoperative ultrasound (IOUS) study in neurosurgery, it is mandatory to accurately plan the surgical approach. The craniotomy has to be large enough to fit the US probe leaving the possibility to direct the US beam on each plan. The surgical cavity must be horizontal in order to be filled by saline solution to allow good acoustic coupling. Another important precaution consists in limiting the use of hemostatic materials because being hyperechoic reduces the field of view.

Once the craniotomy has been completed and the operculum has been removed, the initial US scan is performed through the intact *dura mater*. The probe is placed on the meningeal surface that is continuously irrigated with saline solution to wash away the hyperechoic blood. Prior to contrast-enhanced ultrasound study, a detailed baseline examination is performed with standard B-mode and Doppler imaging. The baseline examination must identify the principal anatomical landmarks and the vascularity of that region. Landmarks recognition is fundamental in order to correctly understand the plan of insonation and structure orientation.

Main landmarks are:

- *Hyperechoic*: skull, vessels walls, choroid plexuses, arachnoid, ependyma, dural fold, brain-lesion interface
- *Hypoechoic*: cerebrospinal fluid, ventricles
- *Isoechoic*: brain parenchyma

Another important task during basal examination is to recognize the lesion, its orientation, relationships with neighboring structure and surrounding vessels [3, 10].

13.2.3 Ultrasound Contrast Agent Preparation

To perform a continuous imaging, second-generation CAs are used. The most used is SonoVue® (Bracco, Italy). It is provided as a lyophilized powder and has to be reconstituted with sterile saline solution (5 ml of NaCl 9 mg/ml) according to the manufacturer recommendations. After reconstitution, UCA is agitated vigorously to obtain a whitish suspension of sulfur hexafluoride MB [5]. UCA (half vial (2.4 ml) for each scan) is then injected trough a peripheral vein, followed by a flush of 10 ml of saline solution.

13.2.4 CEUS Exam

Before dural opening but after the basal scan, the surgeon selects the region of interest and sets the US focus below it. The US modality is switched to contrast-specific imaging mode. This modality reduces the power of insonation to a low-mechanical index (low MI B-mode <0.2) and activates the contrast-specific algorithm; it prevents the MB disruption and allows to visualize only the harmonic signal from UCA. SonoVue (2.4 ml) is injected intravenously followed by a 10 ml of saline flush by anesthesiologist, while surgeon starts the timer and cine-clip recording. Circulating MBs have a half-life of several minutes; this feature allows to follow vessels or to study lesion vascularization with great detail. Moreover during surgery, it is possible to review the cine clip of the CEUS exam, and if this is insufficient, it is possible to repeat CEUS study several times [3].

13.2.5 Limitations

The principal limitation is related to the operator experience with intraoperative US imaging. Specific training in the use of intraoperative CEUS is required.

CEUS is demanding on both theoretical and practical level. It requires a specific knowledge of US physics, US cerebral semeiotics, as well as specific training in CEUS [1, 6].

UCA are approved drugs for diagnostic use in Europe, with some specific contraindications. Patients with severe cardiac insufficiency, right-to-left shunts, severe pulmonary hypertension, uncontrolled systemic hypertension, and adult respiratory distress syndrome should not undergo to the exam [5]. However SonoVue® is a safe drug with almost no side effects, and it does not even require a specific consent [5, 11].

In the matter of surgical limitations, it must be considered that IOUS requires a custom craniotomy to fit the US probe on each orientation. Care must be taken also in using haemostatic materials in order to not reduce the field of view. Furthermore, when performing the US study, it is mandatory to apply only a slight pressure over the neural structures to prevent vessel ruptures or parenchymal contusions [2].

13.3   Clinical Applications in Neurosurgery

Ultrasound contrast agents (UCA) are suspensions of MB of gas encapsulated in a layer of proteins or polymers. The pharmacokinetic of MB is directly related to their mean diameter of 5 μm. Injected through a peripheral vein, MB can pass in smallest capillaries and across the lung, allowing imaging of arterial, capillary, and venous districts. MBs behave as echo-enhancers: they were used at the beginning to enhance Doppler imaging. Doppler imaging permits to visualize the vascular tree, but it is not possible to study in detail and simultaneously arterial and venous flows and so tumor and organ perfusion [12]. CEUS is the only IOUS modality permitting to study all the vascular districts without the need to set pulse repetition frequency, gain, or multiple parameters and without the limitations of low temporal resolution and angle dependency.

One main aspect of UCA in brain application is that they behave as purely intravascular contrast agent because of the dimensions that do not permit to diffuse in the interstitial space [1–3, 6, 13]. The brain has a terminal circulation sustained by multiple arteries, and it demonstrates an arterial, a parenchymal, and a venous phase.

The normal lobar parenchyma does not have a strong enhancement, except for the basal ganglia (Fig. 13.1).

In view of this, two major applications of CEUS in neurosurgery are actually under investigation (Fig. 13.2):

• Intraoperative evaluation of neoplastic lesions
• Angiosonography

13.3.1 Intraoperative Evaluation of Neoplastic Lesions

Over the years, CEUS has proven to be a reliable solution to detect and characterize focal lesions in liver and many other organs. However, only few studies have been published so far in oncological neurosurgery [3, 8, 14–17], and today this technique is not widespread.

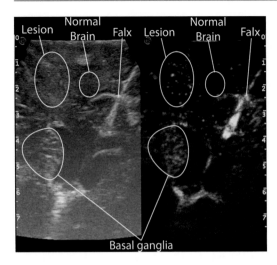

Fig. 13.1 Normal brain parenchyma enhancement. Coronal CEUS scan in a case of a right frontal low-grade glioma. Normal parenchyma does not show any contrast enhancement, while basal ganglia typically show. Lower-grade gliomas usually do not demonstrate a strong contrast enhancement

Our group has been using UCA to perform CEUS for years and has published three studies concerning the topic [2, 3, 8]. We have observed that CEUS with SonoVue® is capable to highlight tumor parenchyma and tumor-brain interface with great accuracy in most tumors. Especially in those tumors that have bad defined border, we have observed that CEUS can show tumor extension with great contrast to healthy edematous brain (Fig. 13.3).

This is due to the pharmacokinetics of UCA that behaves as a purely intravascular contrast agent. The degree of contrast enhancement (CE) post UCA injection is related to the density and distribution of capillaries in the region of interest. The differentiation between tumoral and healthy tissue is based on the tumor enhancement post-contrast injection, that is due to the abnormal density of capillaries in the pathological tissue (Fig. 13.3). This feature permits also to identify

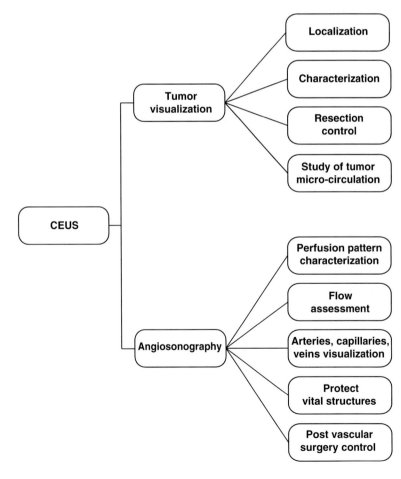

Fig. 13.2 Schematic representation of CEUS applications in neurosurgery

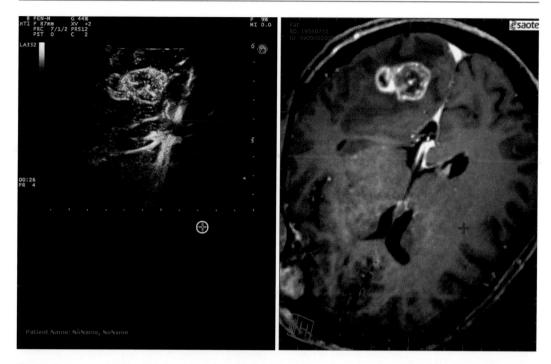

Fig. 13.3 Tumor visualization. Screenshot of navigated IOUS in a case of right parieto-occipital metastasis; axial CEUS scan is shown together with coplanar preoperative MRI. CEUS is able to highlight the lesion margins

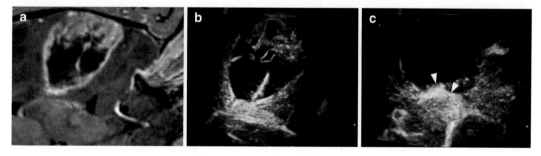

Fig. 13.4 Resection control. Axial CEUS scan in a case of left temporal high-grade glioma. (**a**) Preoperative MRI. (**b**) Pre-resection CEUS scan. (**c**) After partial resection, CEUS shows the residual tumor mass (*arrowheads*)

the more active/viable and the necrotic or cystic areas within the tumor. For example, in glioma surgery, CEUS is capable to differentiate low- and high-grade gliomas and in specific cases can show anaplastic foci in otherwise considered low-grade tumors [8]. On the other hand, those lesions not metabolically active, like dermoid or epidermoid cysts, abscess, and radionecrosis, show no CE, permitting the differential diagnosis between these entity and other necrotic/cystic lesions [3].

Being a tomographic imaging able to discriminate healthy brain and tumor, CEUS allows to repeatedly assess the degree of tumor removal and the residual volume also in region not already exposed (Figs. 13.4 and 13.5).

Furthermore, CEUS, being real time, permits to study all the dynamics of UCA in the tumor. Differently from other contrast-enhanced imaging techniques as computed tomography or magnetic resonance imaging, CEUS shows the enhancement behavior from UCA arrival to the

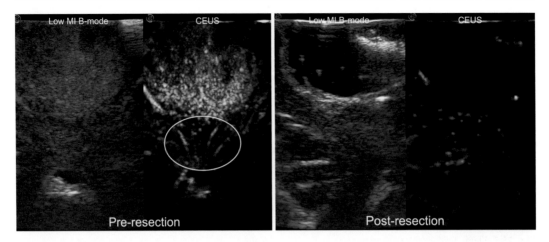

Fig. 13.5 Resection control. CEUS scan in a case of left parietal high-grade glioma. Pre-resection image show the tumor mass and the drainage system toward the ventricle (*circle*). Post-resection image show no contrast enhancement and the disappearance of drainage system

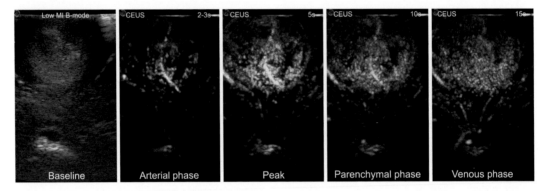

Fig. 13.6 Contrast enhancement phases. CEUS scan in a case of left parietal high-grade glioma. In arterial phase, the main feeders are recognizable. In peak and parenchy- mal phase, it is possible to differentiate more viable and cystic/necrotic areas. In venous phase, multiple small draining veins toward the ventricle are visible

washout phase (Fig. 13.6). For this reason, the CE is subdivided in three main phases:

- Arterial
- Parenchymal
- Venous

This aspect is extremely relevant in case of highly vascularized tumors as meningiomas, in which the possibility to find also deep feeders permits to rapidly devascularize the tumour, reducing the bleeding entity and the surgical complexity (Fig. 13.7).

Moreover, each pathological entity shows a specific CE pattern, in virtue of a specific vascu-

lar organization of afferent vessels, capillaries, and drainage veins.

13.3.2 Contrast Enhancement Pattern

Glioblastomas (GBM) demonstrate a brief CE (20–30 s after UCA injection) characterized by rapid arterial phase (2–3 s), CE peak at 3–5 s, and disordered dynamics of microbubbles within the lesion (Fig. 13.6). In most cases, the arterial feeders are clearly visible, together with many macro-vessels within the lesion and a typical peripheral enhancement that moves centripe-

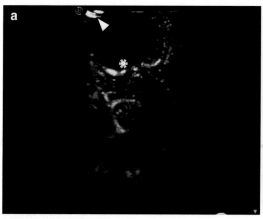
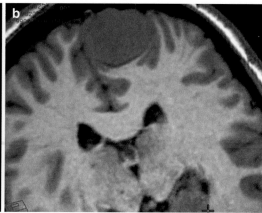

Fig. 13.7 Dural feeders in meningioma surgery. Axial CEUS scan in a case of parasagittal meningioma. (**a**) CEUS scan after dural coagulation. (**b**) Coplanar navigated preoperative MRI. CEUS demonstrates that the main feeders were from the exposed dura mater at the con-vexity: after its coagulation, the tumor shows a little contrast enhancement on the deeper capsule (*asterisk*). The presence of microbubbles in the superior sagittal sinus proves its patency (*arrowhead*)

tally. The parenchymal phase has an irregular and heterogeneous CE pattern with both nodular high-contrast dense areas and hypo-/non-perfused necrotic-cystic areas surrounded by a ring-like enhancement. Also the venous phase is rapid (5–10 s), through a diffuse drainage system and multiple medullary veins directed to the periventricular zone (Figs. 13.5 and 13.6).

Anaplastic gliomas (ANA) usually have a slower arterial phase compared to GBMs (10 s) and a CE peak at approximately 15 s after UCA arrival. The MB transit is less chaotic with the venous phase delayed at 20–25 s. Arterial supplier and venous drainage are less recognizable than in GBMs. ANAs normally have an initial mild and more homogeneous CE compared to GBMs, followed by a reinforcement during the parenchymal phase. In some cases, few small hypoperfused areas are identifiable together with scattered areas of higher CE. The boundaries of the tumor are less distinguishable than in GBMs.

Low-grade gliomas (LGG) show a longer arterial phase (up to 15 s) if compared to ANAs and GBMs and a CE peak at around 20 s. The transit of the MB appears quite regular with a venous phase after 30 s. Arterial supply is not always clear, as well as the venous drainage. LGGs have a soft CE post UCA injection compared to brain parenchyma, and the tumor parenchymal phase is homogeneous. No intralesional vessels are observable.

Meningiomas show a strong and rapid CE; arterial phase of 5–10 s with higher CE peaks in higher grades. CE moves centripetally from the dural attachment with a CE pattern in parenchymal phase strong and homogeneous. The venous phase is delayed (30 s), and venous drainage system is visible. Intralesional major vessels are recognizable only in grade II and III meningiomas, which also exhibited more heterogeneous pattern with hypodense/necrotic areas within the lesion. Tumor margins are always clearly detectable.

Ependymomas are characterized by a rapid arterial phase (5 s) and a CE peak at 5–10 s. The arterial supply is distinguishable and CE moves centripetally, with some macro-vessels within the lesion. The venous phase occurs at 20–25 s, through a diffuse drainage system around the lesion. During parenchymal phase, the CE pattern is irregular and heterogeneous homogeneous areas alternating with hypoperfused cystic areas.

Pituitary adenomas have a brief arterial phase (10 s) and a delayed CE peak at 30 s. Arterial feeders are not visible, as well as the veins, and the CE pattern is quite regular and homogeneous. No vessels inside the tumor are visible.

Parenchymal phase is persistent with a slow venous phase (>40 s).

Craniopharyngiomas have a slow arterial phase (40–50 s) and a delayed CE peak at 80 s. The CE pattern is heterogeneous, and feeding and draining vessels are not detectable. No vessels are recognizable inside the lesion. The parenchymal phase is persistent with a slow venous phase (100 s).

Hemangioblastomas display a rapid arterial phase (5–10 s) and CE peak. CE is intense with a centripetal progression. The CE pattern shows homogeneous parenchymal areas together with hypoperfused regions. No major vessels are visible within the lesion. The venous phase is delayed up to 30 s.

Metastases, in most cases, show a rapid and fast arterial phase (2–3 s) and CE peak (at 5–10 s). The arterial feeders are usually visible with many macro-vessels within the lesion. CE progress centripetally, and it is persistent with a slow venous phase (30 s). The drainage system is not visible. CE in metastases is typically strong and intense with an irregular pattern composed of high-contrast dense areas, macro-vessels, and hypo-/non-perfused necrotic/cystic areas. Tumor borders are commonly identifiable after CE.

Epidermoid/dermoid cysts, abscess, radionecrosis are not metabolically active and do not show any CE, not having a specialized vascularization.

In general, CEUS is able to highlight different brain lesions, both intra- and extra-axial, as compared to standard B-mode imaging.

Relying on our preliminary data, CEUS has the ability to depict lesions such as high-grade gliomas with a detailed morphology superimposable to that of T1-weighted contrast-enhanced MRI (Fig. 13.4). Therefore, CEUS is highly desirable in those cases when the standard B-mode is not able to differentiate between the lesion and brain tissue (Fig. 13.3).

Moreover, as it has been shown by our group, it also allows a real-time characterization of different histotype. Furthermore, CEUS permits to visualize tumor remnants after resection, partially overcoming the problems due to artifacts (Figs. 13.4 and 13.5).

CEUS offers also valuable biological information regarding tumor perfusion, as well as tumor vascularization: the possibility to visualize afferent and efferent vessels allows to localize them in the surgical field, thus possibly changing the surgical strategy for tumor removal (Fig. 13.7)

13.4 Angiosonography

Even though the main studied application of CEUS is cerebral tumor surgery, the second most relevant is the study of vascular tree when dealing with vessels [7, 16] (Fig. 13.2).

CEUS is a harmonic imaging modality that depicts only the echo signal from the MBs that measuring 2–6 μm can distribute exclusively inside the vascular tree.

In virtue of their dimensions, MB can pass in arteries, veins, and also capillaries. This feature permits to study not only the principal vessels but also the general perfusion pattern of the region or lesion without the need to set multiple parameters as for Doppler imaging [12]. Moreover, CEUS, being an echo-tomographic representation allows to study vessels in depth, not already surgically exposed, as requested, for example, by fluorescence-guided surgery [7] (Figs. 13.8, 13.9, and 13.10).

These aspects together with the excellent spatial and temporal resolution and repeatability of CEUS make possible to localize and follow the entire course of a vessel of interest simply by tilting the probe.

Vessels localization is only the first result of CEUS examination. Through a visual qualitative evaluation of the direction and velocity of MB movements and observing the intensity of signal, it is possible to establish the flow direction and entity.

In oncological surgery, CEUS is useful to identify and locate shifted or encased main vascular structures, feeding and draining systems, leading tumor resection and assisting vessels dissection [2, 7] (Figs. 13.7, 13.8, and 13.9). Ultimately CEUS aids to preserve vital structures or to reduce the bleeding entity by sacrificing the feeding arteries (Figs. 13.7 and 13.10).

In vascular surgery, CEUS is applicable when coping with aneurysms, arteriovenous malformations (AVM), and in general every time that a vessel undergoes a prolonged manipulation (Figs. 13.8, 13.9, and 13.10).

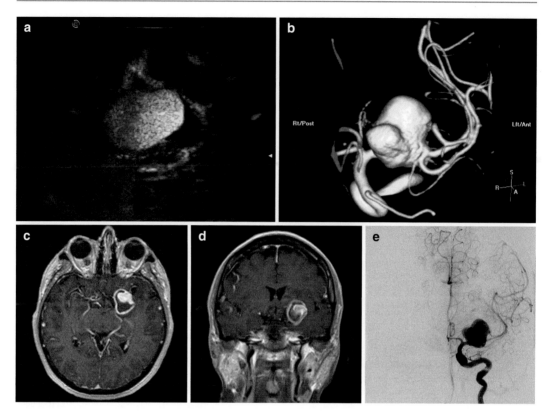

Fig. 13.8 Angiosonography in aneurysm surgery. (**a**) CEUS scan in a case of left middle cerebral artery bifurcation aneurysm. (**b**) 3D angiography reconstruction. (**c, d**) Preoperative MRI. (**e**) Angiography. The aneurysm is partially thrombosed; indeed, CEUS shows inhomogeneous contrast distribution in the *sac*. The angiosonography highlights *sac* orientation and its relationships to the middle cerebral artery bifurcation

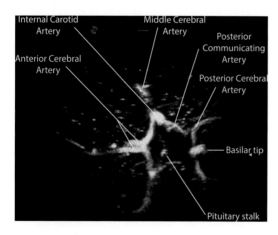

Fig. 13.9 Angiosonography of the circle of Willis in a case of frontotemporal low-grade glioma

In AVM surgery, CEUS allows to visualize the nidus as well as feeding and draining vessels and permits to be aware of any residual mass prior to exposure [7, 16]. During resection, it is of help in visualizing arterial feeders when progressively dissecting the nidus. After resection, CEUS can be repeated to check the cavity for residual AVM (Fig. 13.10).

When dealing with aneurysms, CEUS makes possible to evaluate sac morphology and orientation in regard of main proximal and distal vessels [7, 16] (Fig. 13.8), prior to direct exposure. After clipping the aneurysm, CEUS allows to assess distal flow, also comparing the real-time imaging to pre-clipping situation.

In addition to direct visualization during vascular surgery procedure, CEUS permits to perform a control in order to study the obtained effects: in fact in general, after prolonged manipulation of a vessel, the presence of MBs' flow certifies its patency.

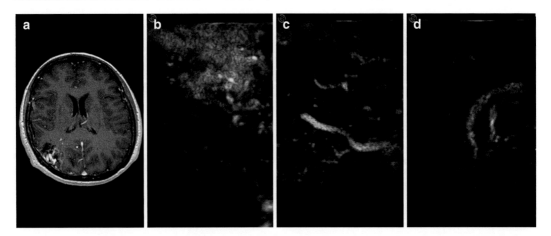

Fig. 13.10 Angiosonography in a case of right parietal arteriovenous malformation. (**a**) Preoperative MRI. (**b**) CEUS scan of the nidus. (**c**) CEUS scan of the principal arterial feeders. (**d**) CEUS scan of the drainage system toward the ventricle

References

1. Piscaglia F, Nolsoe C, Dietrich CF, Cosgrove DO, Gilja OH, Bachmann Nielsen M, Albrecht T, Barozzi L, Bertolotto M, Catalano O, Claudon M, Clevert DA, Correas JM, D'Onofrio M, Drudi FM, Eyding J, Giovannini M, Hocke M, Ignee A, Jung EM, Klauser AS, Lassau N, Leen E, Mathis G, Saftoiu A, Seidel G, Sidhu PS, ter Haar G, Timmerman D, Weskott HP (2012) The EFSUMB Guidelines and Recommendations on the Clinical Practice of Contrast Enhanced Ultrasound (CEUS): update 2011 on non-hepatic applications. Ultraschall Med (Stuttgart, Germany: 1980) 33(1):33–59. doi:10.1055/s-0031-1281676

2. Prada F, Del Bene M, Moiraghi A, Casali C, Legnani FG, Saladino A, Perin A, Vetrano IG, Mattei L, Richetta C, Saini M, DiMeco F (2015) From grey scale B-mode to elastosonography: multimodal ultrasound imaging in meningioma surgery—pictorial essay and literature review. BioMed Res Int 2015:13. doi:10.1155/2015/925729

3. Prada F, Perin A, Martegani A, Aiani L, Solbiati L, Lamperti M, Casali C, Legnani F, Mattei L, Saladino A, Saini M, DiMeco F (2014) Intraoperative contrast-enhanced ultrasound for brain tumor surgery. Neurosurgery 74(5):542–552. doi:10.1227/neu.0000000000000301; discussion 552

4. Smirniotopoulos JG, Murphy FM, Rushing EJ, Rees JH, Schroeder JW (2007) Patterns of contrast enhancement in the brain and meninges. RadioGraphics 27(2):525–551. doi:10.1148/rg.272065155

5. EMA (2014) SonoVue -EMEA/H/C/000303 -II/0025. http://www.ema.europa.eu/ema/index.jsp?

6. Claudon M, Dietrich CF, Choi BI, Cosgrove DO, Kudo M, Nolsoe CP, Piscaglia F, Wilson SR, Barr RG, Chammas MC, Chaubal NG, Chen MH, Clevert DA, Correas JM, Ding H, Forsberg F, Fowlkes JB, Gibson RN, Goldberg BB, Lassau N, Leen EL, Mattrey RF, Moriyasu F, Solbiati L, Weskott HP, Xu HX (2013) Guidelines and good clinical practice recommendations for contrast enhanced ultrasound (CEUS) in the liver – update 2012: a WFUMB-EFSUMB initiative in cooperation with representatives of AFSUMB, AIUM, ASUM, FLAUS and ICUS. Ultraschall Med (Stuttgart, Germany: 1980) 34(1):11–29. doi:10.1055/s-0032-1325499

7. Prada F, Del Bene M, Saini M, Ferroli P, DiMeco F (2015) Intraoperative cerebral angiosonography with ultrasound contrast agents: how I do it. Acta Neurochir 157(6):1025–1029. doi:10.1007/s00701-015-2412-x

8. Prada F, Mattei L, Del Bene M, Aiani L, Saini M, Casali C, Filippini A, Legnani FG, Perin A, Saladino A, Vetrano IG, Solbiati L, Martegani A, DiMeco F (2014) Intraoperative cerebral glioma characterization with contrast enhanced ultrasound. BioMed Res Int 2014:9. doi:10.1155/2014/484261

9. van Leyen K, Klotzsch C, Harrer JU (2011) Brain tumor imaging with transcranial sonography: state of the art and review of the literature. Ultraschall Med (Stuttgart, Germany: 1980) 32(6):572–581. doi:10.1055/s-0031-1273443

10. Prada F, Del Bene M, Mattei L, Lodigiani L, DeBeni S, Kolev V, Vetrano I, Solbiati L, Sakas G, DiMeco F (2014) Preoperative magnetic resonance and intraoperative ultrasound fusion imaging for real-time neuronavigation in brain tumor surgery. Ultraschall Med (Stuttgart, Germany: 1980). doi:10.1055/s-0034-1385347

11. Piscaglia F, Bolondi L (2006) The safety of Sonovue in abdominal applications: retrospective analysis of 23188 investigations. Ultrasound Med Biol 32(9):1369–1375. doi:10.1016/j.ultrasmedbio.2006.05.031

12. Gibbs V, Cole D, Sassano A (2009) Ultrasound physics and technology. Elsevier, Churchill Livingstone

13. Quaia E (2011) Assessment of tissue perfusion by contrast-enhanced ultrasound. Eur Radiol 21(3):604–615. doi:10.1007/s00330-010-1965-6

14. Engelhardt M, Hansen C, Eyding J, Wilkening W, Brenke C, Krogias C, Scholz M, Harders A, Ermert H, Schmieder K (2007) Feasibility of contrast-enhanced sonography during resection of cerebral tumours: initial results of a prospective study. Ultrasound Med Biol 33(4):571–575. doi:10.1016/j.ultrasmedbio.2006.10.007

15. He W, Jiang XQ, Wang S, Zhang MZ, Zhao JZ, Liu HZ, Ma J, Xiang DY, Wang LS (2008) Intraoperative contrast-enhanced ultrasound for brain tumors. Clin Imaging 32(6):419–424. doi:10.1016/j.clinimag.2008.05.006

16. Holscher T, Ozgur B, Singel S, Wilkening WG, Mattrey RF, Sang H (2007) Intraoperative ultrasound using phase inversion harmonic imaging: first experiences. Neurosurgery 60(4 Suppl 2):382–386. doi:10.1227/01.neu.0000255379.87840.6e; discussion 386–387

17. Kanno H, Ozawa Y, Sakata K, Sato H, Tanabe Y, Shimizu N, Yamamoto I (2005) Intraoperative power Doppler ultrasonography with a contrast-enhancing agent for intracranial tumors. J Neurosurg 102(2):295–301. doi:10.3171/jns.2005.102.2.0295

Part VI

Elastosonography

Ultrasound Elastography

14

Huan Wee Chan, Jeffrey Bamber, Neil Dorward,
Aabir Chakraborty, and Christopher Uff

14.1   Introduction

Medical practitioners perform palpation as part of their clinical examination to detect any abnormalities. They perform palpation by exerting certain force on the soft tissue with their hands and rely on tactile feedback to assess the response of the soft tissue. Using their knowledge about the stiffness of normal tissue, they determine if the soft tissue they are palpating is normal or abnormal. In essence, they are assessing the amount of soft tissue deformation in response to certain amount of force, which is the definition of Young's modulus given by:

$$E = \frac{\text{Stress}}{\text{Strain}}$$

where E is the Young's modulus, stress is the amount of deformation force applied and strain is the amount of deformation in response to the deformation force. During palpation, medical practitioners invariably apply the same amount of force; thus, they rely on the relative soft tissue strain to detect any abnormalities.

Quasistatic strain elastography (QSE) is the one of the earliest type of elastography described in 1991 by Ophir et al. [1]. This technique uses ultrasound to image the soft tissue before and after applying deformation force. The amount of strain exhibited by the soft tissue is displayed as strain imaging. This is very similar to palpation, except that it has better resolution and higher sensitivity than palpation. This is especially useful in lesions that are situated deep in the soft tissue.

Ultrasound elastography is the name given to ultrasound-based techniques of imaging soft tissue elasticity. Ultrasound images are made up of tiny white granules known as speckles, which are produced by interference of echoes (reflected sound waves) from very small reflectors present in biological tissue. These speckles act as image markers for ultrasound imaging to track during soft tissue deformation. Using high-frequency ultrasound imaging, the motion of the speckles between neighbouring elements can be detected and mapped with high resolution. This forms the basis for ultrasound elastography.

There are several methods of performing such imaging. Generally, they can be divided into qualitative and quantitative elastography. As the

H.W. Chan (✉) • N. Dorward • C. Uff
Victor Horsley Department of Neurosurgery,
The National Hospital for Neurology and
Neurosurgery, Queen Square,
London WC1N 3BG, UK
e-mail: chanhuanwee@gmail.com

J. Bamber
Joint Department of Physics, Institute of Cancer
Research and The Royal Marsden Hospital,
15 Cotswold Road, Sutton SM2 5NG, UK

A. Chakraborty
Wessex Neurological Centre, Southampton
General Hospital, Tremona Road, Southampton
SO16 6YD, UK

© Springer International Publishing Switzerland 2016
F. Prada et al. (eds.), *Intraoperative Ultrasound (IOUS) in Neurosurgery:
From Standard B-mode to Elastosonography*, DOI 10.1007/978-3-319-25268-1_14

name implies, qualitative elastography demonstrates the relative stiffness of one type of soft tissue compared to another. The examples of this type of elastography are QSE, as described above, and acoustic radiation force impulse (ARFI) imaging. On the other hand, quantitative elastography displays the absolute stiffness of the soft tissue being imaged. The absolute stiffness can be displayed as Young's modulus or shear modulus in kilopascal (kPa) unit. The examples of quantitative elastography are shear wave elastography (SWE) and crawling wave imaging.

ARFI imaging utilises focused ultrasound beams emitted by the ultrasound transducer to produce minute deformation of the soft tissue, which is detected by ultrasound imaging [2]. As the stress produced is not uniform, the Young's modulus cannot be determined. Therefore, the resultant strain images are qualitative.

In SWE, focused ultrasound beams are used to cause micromillimetre displacement of the soft tissue to produce shear waves, which travel in the plane perpendicular to the axis of displacement [3]. The speed of the shear waves is related to Young's modulus by the equation:

$$E = 3\rho c^2$$

where E is Young's modulus, ρ is density of soft tissue and c is shear wave speed. Using the same principle as tracking speckle motion, ultrasound imaging is able to produce a map of shear wave speed with relatively high resolution. This is a type of quantitative elastography.

14.2   Clinical Application of Ultrasound Elastography

Ultrasound elastography has been used clinically in different organs. In this section, only clinical application in the liver, breast and thyroid will be discussed.

In the liver, the 'gold standard' for grading liver fibrosis is by doing a liver biopsy [4]. However, this is very invasive and has many potential complications associated with it. Therefore, ultrasound elastography has been employed in the attempt to assess liver fibrosis non-invasively. Transient elastography (TE) is

the first ultrasound elastographic technique for liver [5]. This is a 1D elastographic technique, whereby a low-frequency vibrator, typically 50 Hz, is used to generate shear waves [5].

In the breast, both QSE and SWE are used to reclassifying breast imaging recording and data system (BI-RADS) 4a into 3 and 4b [6], as the management for BI-RADS 3 (probably benign) and BI-RADS 4b (intermediate suspicion of malignancy) are very different, the former not requiring biopsy whereas the latter requiring biopsy. Using Tsukuba 5-point scoring system, in which the amount of stiff tissue in and around the lesion is assessed, QSE was shown to have 71.2 % sensitivity, 96.6 % specificity and 87.4 % accuracy in differentiating benign from malignant lesions when the cut-off point of between 4 and 5 were used [7]. The addition of QSE to B-mode ultrasound has been shown to improve the accuracy of BI-RADS classifications [8]. Using a cut-off value of maximum Young's modulus of 80 kilopascal (kPa), SWE was shown to be able to reclassify BI-RADS 3 and 4a, thus improving the specificity of conventional ultrasound from 61.1 to 78.5 % without adversely affecting the sensitivity in 650 lesions [9].

In the thyroid, QSE and SWE have been used in differentiating benign from malignant nodules. A meta-analysis of 639 nodules demonstrated that QSE had a mean sensitivity and specificity of 92 % and 90 %, respectively, for diagnosing malignancy thyroid nodules [10]. Shear wave speed using SWE has been shown to be higher in malignant nodules compared to benign nodules, but the cut-off maximal have not been consistent [11, 12].

14.3   Intraoperative Ultrasound Elastography in Neurosurgery

Neurosurgeons invariably rely on visual inspection and tactile feedback when performing resection of brain lesions as these lesions usually have different appearance and texture. However, this is very subjective, and neurosurgeons overestimate the extent of resection by three times [13, 14], as the appearance and texture can be very similar to the surrounding brain.

Neuronavigation using preoperative imaging has been employed to improve the extent of resection. In fact, neuronavigation plays a vital role in assisting neurosurgeons in craniotomy planning and surgical approach to the lesion [15]. However, brain shift occurs after craniotomy and dural opening. If the intracranial pressure is high prior to craniotomy, the brain and the lesion bulge towards the craniotomy site. Conversely, if the intracranial pressure is normal or low prior to craniotomy, the whole brain including the lesion will sink away from the craniotomy site. This is further exacerbated by dural opening, where drainage of cerebrospinal fluid (CSF) and gravity will cause further shift. It was shown that the mean shift of the cortex is 4.6 mm after dural opening and 6.7 mm after tumour resection [16]. Therefore, although neuronavigation helps with craniotomy planning and surgical approach, it is not very accurate in determining the extent of resection.

Intraoperative ultrasound (IOUS) in neurosurgery has been used since the 1980s [17]. However, the application of IOUS in neurosurgery is limited due to the low-quality images, unfamiliarity of ultrasound among neurosurgeons and user-dependent variability in image interpretation. With the advancement in image processing and computer technology, the quality of ultrasound images has improved significantly. The improvement in image quality, combined with the capability of co-registering the ultrasound transducer with neuronavigation, has revived the use of IOUS in neurosurgery [18]. Not only is IOUS easy to set up and relatively low cost, it also provides real-time imaging of brain structures during surgery. With no ionising radiation risk, IOUS can be used as many times as the neurosurgeon requires to guide resection of brain lesion.

Whereas IOUS demonstrates the structural anatomy of the brain during surgery, ultrasound elastography reveals the elasticity of the brain lesion to be resected without direct palpation of the lesion. This will provide neurosurgeons with additional information to facilitate maximal extent of resection and prevent neurological deterioration. As the majority of brain lesions are stiffer than surrounding brain, neurosurgeons usually know when they are resecting the lesions.

However, in some cases where the lesions are softer than surrounding brain, neurosurgeons might compromise patient safety if excessive force is used to resect these lesions. Additionally, as neurosurgeons normally encounter lesions stiffer than brain, these softer lesions might be missed. Some lesions even have similar stiffness to surrounding brain, making it even more difficult for neurosurgeons to resect them safely. These lesions, however, will be difficult to visualise even with ultrasound elastography. Therefore, neurosurgeons will rely on other information such as hyperintensity on MRI, hyperechogenicity on IOUS and different visual appearance of such lesions to assist them during surgery.

Ultrasound elastography is a relatively new technique and a research tool in neurosurgery. This chapter will describe the different types of ultrasound elastography used in neurosurgery intraoperatively.

14.3.1 Types of Intraoperative Ultrasound Elastography in Neurosurgery

There are different types of ultrasound elastography being researched in neurosurgery:

1. Quasistatic strain elastography
2. Vibrography
3. Slip elastography
4. Shear wave elastography

The first three types of elastography listed above are qualitative elastography and require external force to be applied in order to create elasticity maps, called elastograms. The last type of elastography above is quantitative elastography and does not require external force application.

14.3.2 Quasistatic Strain Elastography

QSE is one of the earliest types of elastography, first described by Ophir et al. [1]. As described in the previous chapter, QSE is performed by applying an external force to deform the soft tissue being scanned. The amount of deformation will depend on the elasticity of the lesion. In response to the same external force, the softer lesion will deform more than the surrounding brain while the harder lesion less than the surrounding brain. As the external force applied is not uniform, the resultant elastograms are qualitative.

The first intraoperative QSE in neurosurgery was described by Chakraborty et al. [19, 20], which demonstrated the biomechanical properties of the brain tumour and brain-tumour interface (Fig. 14.1). The QSE employed by this group requires freehand external force applica-

tion with an extended footplate attached to the ultrasound transducer to allow a more uniform deformation. The elastograms were created offline, i.e. at a later time after the images were acquired, as the computer technology at the time was not fast enough for real-time image processing. Therefore, this precluded the real-time application of QSE in guiding resection.

Selbekk et al. [21, 22] demonstrated that it is feasible to perform QSE by holding the ultrasound transducer static on the brain surface to allow brain pulsation to create deformation in the brain and the lesion. The same group showed that the elastograms obtained through this method was

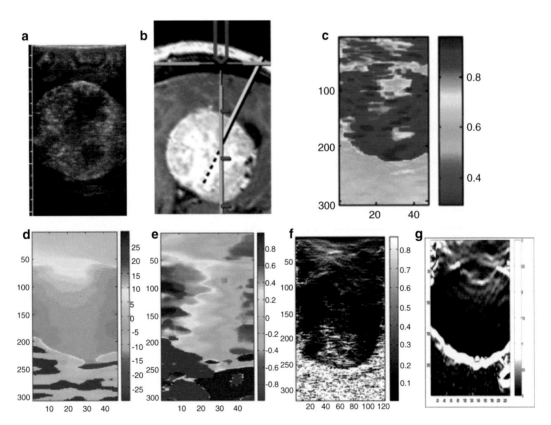

Fig. 14.1 Intraoperative QSE of a patient with meningioma. The ultrasound B-mode image (**a**) and the corresponding MRI image on the Stealth neuronavigation system (**b**). (**c**) Correlation coefficient image, which measures the quality of the elastograms; the values from within the tumour are mostly greater than 0.9, with 1 being perfect correlation. (**d**, **e**) are axial and lateral displacement images, respectively; displacement images are produced by tracking the displacement of each individual speckle. Lateral displacement image (**e**) has poorer quality compared to axial displacement image (**d**). Greyscale elastogram with external compression (**g**) demonstrated the slip boundary better than the elastogram with no external compression (**f**) (Reproduced from Chakraborty et al. [20])

capable of exhibiting better brain-tumour contrast than B-mode ultrasound [23]. This method of QSE was still processed offline. This further paved the way for the application of QSE in sensitive nervous tissue such as the spinal cord, as demonstrated in a PhD thesis by Uff [24]. The latter QSE was performed using an ultrasound scanner capable of producing real-time elastograms.

Uff et al. [25] showed that it is feasible to perform real-time intraoperative QSE in neurosurgery to demonstrate the biomechanical properties of brain tumours and characterise slip brain-tumour interface (Figs. 14.2 and 14.3). In his PhD thesis, Uff [24] demonstrated that it was possible to characterise slip brain-tumour interface with 2D and 3D QSE, where the latter produces less elevational decorrelation. Figures 14.4 and 14.5 illustrate the 2D and 3D QSE in characterising slip brain-tumour interface, respectively. Furthermore, in the same PhD thesis, Uff [24] showed that QSE was capable of demonstrating

epileptogenic lesions, including those which are not visible on MRI (Fig. 14.6).

14.3.3 Vibrography

Vibrography is a technique described by Pesavento et al. [26], where the strain produced is almost quasistatic by using very low-frequency vibration and very slow compression. Without going into the details of physics behind this technique, using phase root seeking algorithm, this technique was shown to decrease computational cost and improve image quality. Therefore, this allowed the generation of real-time elastograms using the computer technology at the time.

Scholz et al. [27] demonstrated the feasibility of this technique in visualising brain tumour intraoperatively. Later on, the same group [28] showed the capability of this technique to guide

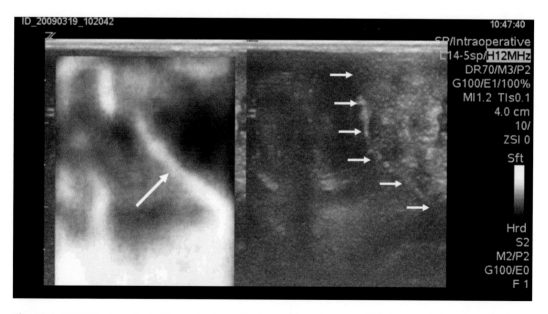

Fig. 14.2 2D QSE of a patient with meningioma. Strain elastogram (*left*) and the corresponding ultrasound B-mode (*right*) of the stiff meningioma with a slip tumour-brain boundary. The *short white arrows* on B-mode (*right*) indicate the boundary between the meningioma in the upper right corner of the image and the surrounding brain. The *long white arrow* on strain elastogram (*right*) indicates high strain at the boundary, suggestive of a mobile boundary (Reproduced from Uff [24])

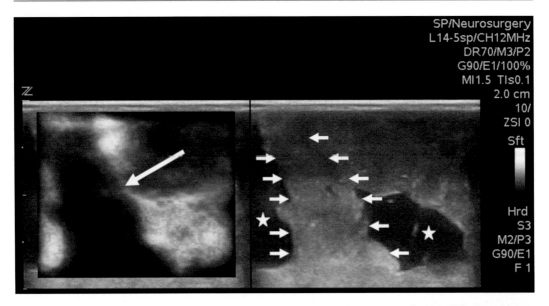

Fig. 14.3 2D QSE of a patient with epidermoid cyst. Strain elastogram (*left*) and the corresponding ultrasound B-mode (*right*) of the stiff epidermoid cyst. The *short arrows* on ultrasound B-mode (*right*) outline the epider-moid cyst, while the *white stars* on either side of the echo-free regions are fluid within the fourth ventricle. The *long white arrows* on strain elastogram (*left*) indicate the high strain at the boundary (Reproduced from Uff [24])

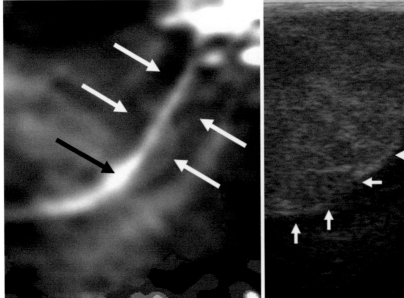

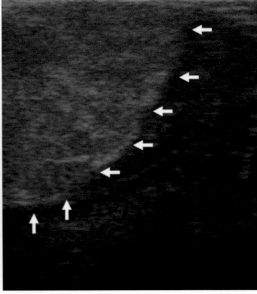

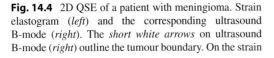

Fig. 14.4 2D QSE of a patient with meningioma. Strain elastogram (*left*) and the corresponding ultrasound B-mode (*right*). The *short white arrows* on ultrasound B-mode (*right*) outline the tumour boundary. On the strain elastogram (*left*), the *black arrow* indicates high strain at the boundary while the *long white arrows* indicate strain heterogeneity on either side of the boundary (Reproduced from Uff [24])

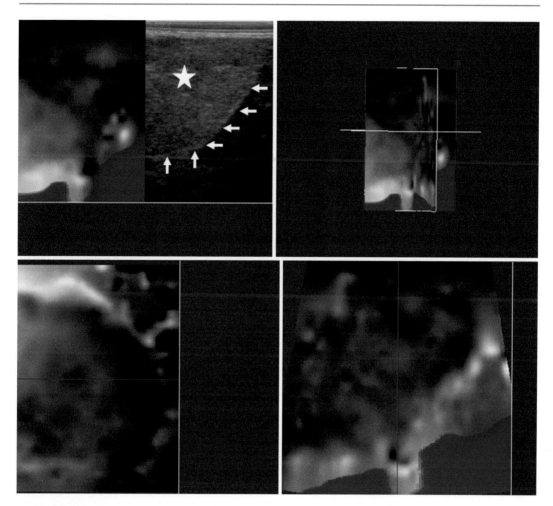

Fig. 14.5 3D QSE of a patient with meningioma, which was imaged with the Diasus scanner in 3D using the multiple volume acquisition method. 2D strain elastogram and the corresponding ultrasound B-mode in the *top left image*. C-plane of the axial elastogram (*bottom left*) is the compound plane in the elevational direction of the axial elastogram. Elevational plane elastogram (*bottom right*) is the strain produced in the elevational direction by the axial force. The *top right image* is the 3D orthogonal slices of the elastogram. The meningioma is the hyperechoic region in the upper left part of the B-mode (*white star*), and its boundary is outlined the *white arrows* (pointing towards the tumour) (Reproduced from Uff [24])

brain tumour resection with the ability to perform vibrography at different stages of brain tumour resection.

14.3.4 Slip Elastography

Slip elastography is a term coined by Chakraborty [29] and Chakraborty et al. [30] to describe the use of elastography to quantify the external force required to create slip brain-tumour interface. Figure 14.7 illustrates the phantom study performed to quantify the force required to cause the slip at different angles. In his PhD thesis, Chakraborty [29] showed the feasibility of this technique in brain tumour resection to quantify the force required to create slip brain-tumour interface in vivo. Figures 14.8, 14.9 and 14.10

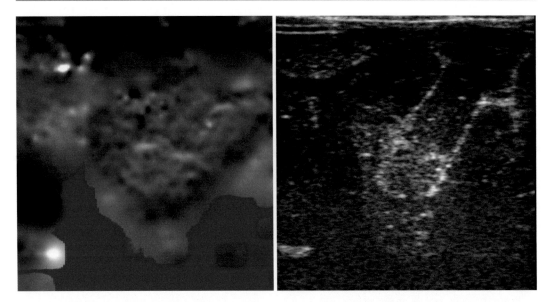

Fig. 14.6 This is an example of a MRI-negative epilepsy case, in which an intraoperative QSE acquisition was performed. Axial strain image (*left*) and the corresponding B-mode (*right*). The epileptogenic lesion was clearly demonstrated on QSE while it was subtle on ultrasound B-mode (Reproduced from Uff [24])

illustrate the use of slip elastography in demonstrating an obvious slip tumour-brain boundary, a cleavage plane in a non-slip tumour-brain boundary and an absent cleavage plane, respectively.

14.3.5 Shear Wave Elastography

Shear wave elastography (SWE) is a quantitative elastography developed by Bercoff et al. [3], which utilises cutting-edge technology of ultra-fast plane wave imaging. A few micromillimetre (μm) displacement is created by highly focused ultrasound beam, i.e. acoustic radiation force, emitted by the ultrasound transducer, to produce shear waves that propagate in the direction perpendicular to the direction of the acoustic radiation force. The shear waves are imaged, and the speed is estimated by the use of ultrafast plane wave imaging.

The first intraoperative SWE in neurosurgery was demonstrated by Uff [24], where he showed that it was feasible to perform intraoperative SWE in brain tumour and epileptogenic lesions (Figs. 14.11 and 14.12, respectively). This paved the way for further research using SWE to verifying the surgical assessment and SWE measurements in brain tumours [31] (Figs. 14.13 and 14.14) and epileptogenic lesions [31, 32] (Fig. 14.15).

Some epileptogenic lesions are not demonstrated clearly on MRI, especially when they are developmental abnormalities such as focal cortical dysplasia and dysembryoplastic neuroepithelial tumour. However, they usually have different elasticity compared to surrounding brain [32]. Chan et al. [33] demonstrated that SWE was capable to detecting MRI-negative epileptogenic lesions with electrophysiological and histological confirmation, including a case report [34] (Fig. 14.16).

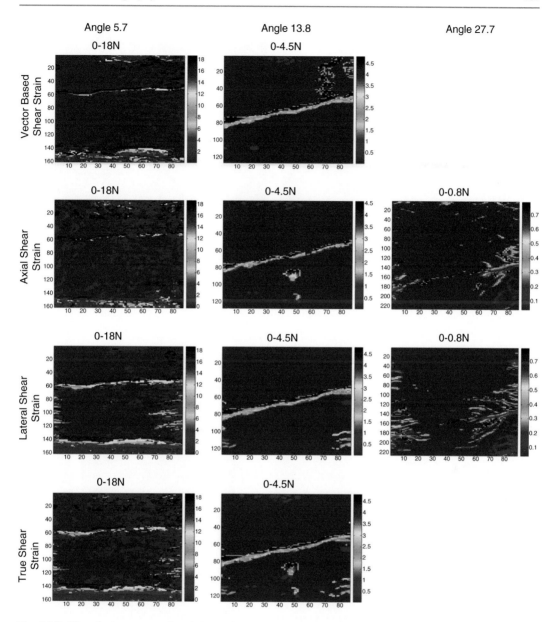

Fig. 14.7 Slip elastograms produced from phantoms with slip boundary angles of 5.7°, 13.8° and 27.7° using the four shear strain estimators tested. Force values are in Newtons, and the range on the colour bar is depicted above each image. The quality of the elastograms pro- duced at angle 27.7° contained a great deal of artefact, so the slip boundary is not clearly seen, and that is why only the lateral and axial shear strain estimators are included (Reproduced from Chakraborty et al. [30])

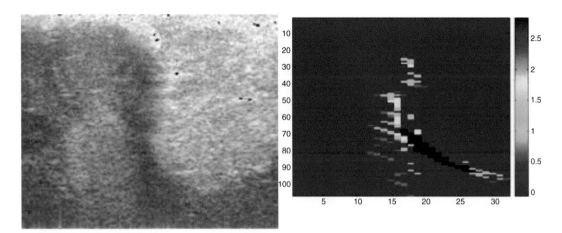

Fig. 14.8 Slip elastography of a patient with meningioma. Ultrasound B-mode (*left*) and the corresponding slip elastogram (*right*). The slip elastogram demonstrates an obvious slip boundary between tumour and brain (Reproduced from Chakraborty [29])

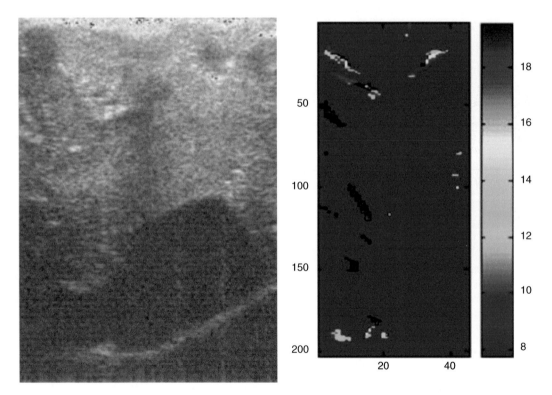

Fig. 14.9 Slip elastography of a patient with glioblastoma multiforme. Ultrasound B-mode (*left*) with the corresponding slip elastogram (*right*). The slip elastogram demonstrated that the tumour was adherent to brain but identified a cleavage plane in the brain-tumour boundary (Reproduced from Chakraborty [29])

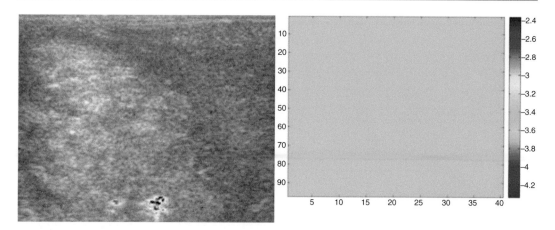

Fig. 14.10 Slip elastography of a patient with glioblastoma multiforme. Ultrasound B-mode (*left*) with the corresponding slip elastogram (*right*). The slip elastogram demonstrated an absence of slip boundary (Reproduced from Chakraborty [29])

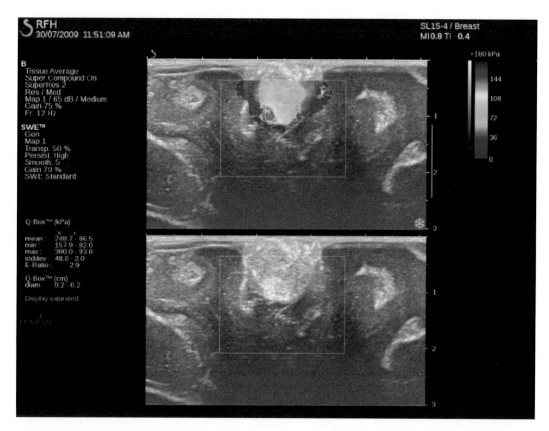

Fig. 14.11 SWE of a patient with a stiff meningioma. The ultrasound B-mode with SWE overlay (*top*) and the same plain ultrasound B-mode (*bottom*) (Reproduced from Uff [24])

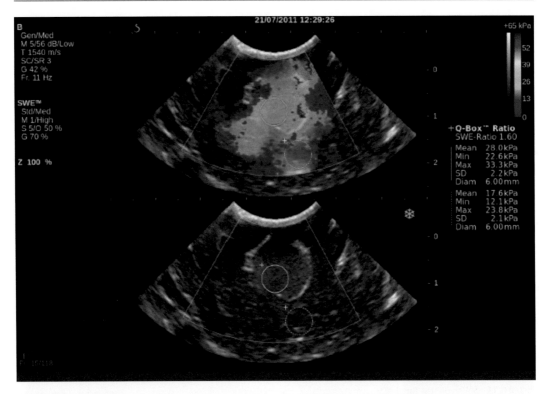

Fig. 14.12 SWE of a patient with focal cortical dysplasia. Ultrasound B-mode with SWE overlay (*top*) and the same plain ultrasound B-mode (*bottom*). The lesion is stiffer than brain (Reproduced from Uff [24])

Conclusions

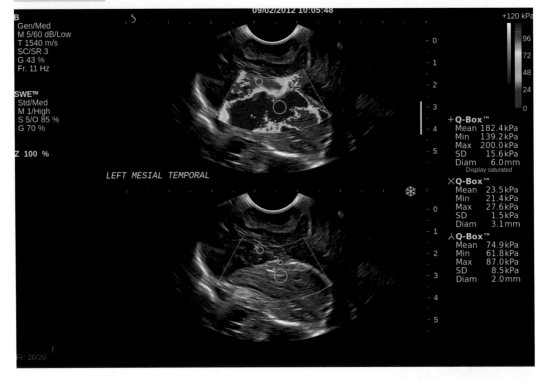

Fig. 14.13 SWE of a patient with medial temporal epidermoid cyst, which was stiffer than normal brain. Ultrasound B-mode with SWE overlay (*top*) and the same plain ultrasound B-mode (*bottom*). This lesion was clearly demonstrated on both SWE and ultrasound B-mode (Adapted from Chan et al. [31])

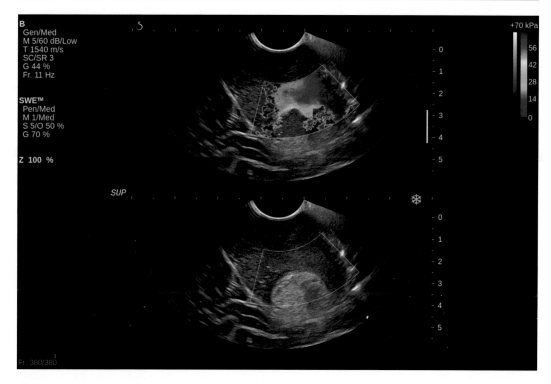

Fig. 14.14 SWE of a patient with cerebellar atypical teratoid rhabdoid tumour, which was found to be extremely stiff during resection. Ultrasound B-mode with SWE overlay (*top*) and the corresponding plain ultrasound B-mode (*bottom*). The lesion was clearly demonstrated in both SWE and ultrasound B-mode (Adapted from Chan [35])

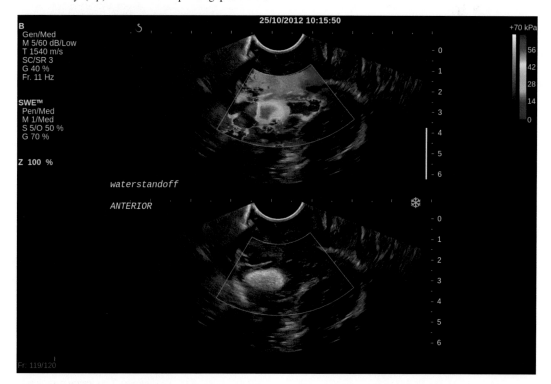

Fig. 14.15 SWE of a patient with a medial temporal dysembryoplastic neuroepithelial tumour. Ultrasound B-mode with SWE overlay (*top*) and the same plain ultrasound B-mode (*bottom*). On the elastogram, the tumour was softer than brain. This was confirmed by surgical assessment during resection of the tumour (Adapted from Chan et al. [32])

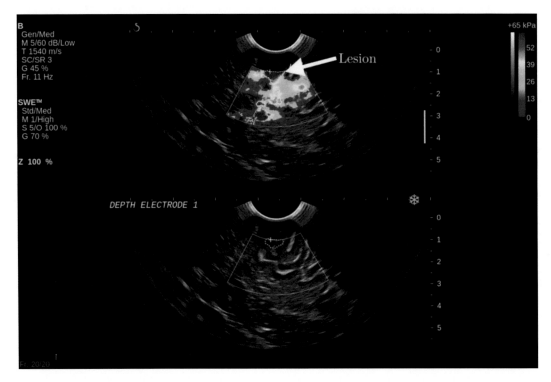

Fig. 14.16 SWE of a patient with MRI-negative focal cortical dysplasia. Ultrasound B-mode with SWE overlay (*top*) and the same plain ultrasound B-mode (*bottom*). The elastogram demonstrated the stiff lesion, which was absent on MRI and ultrasound B-mode. The finding was consistent with surgical assessment of the lesion. The deeper stiff region at 3 cm depth is due white matter anisotropy (Adapted from Chan et al. [34])

Ultrasound elastography is an imaging technique that maps tissue elasticity in real time. When used in neurosurgery as an intraoperative adjunct, ultrasound elastography informs the neurosurgeon the biomechanical properties of the region of surgical exposure, including the surrounding brain, the brain-lesion boundary and the lesion. As brain lesions invariably have different biomechanical properties compared to normal brain, ultrasound elastography can also visualise lesions that are not clearly visible on other imaging modalities. Therefore, ultrasound elastography is a useful intraoperative adjunct that can help guide resection by identification of surgical plane and visualising obscure lesions. When used with other intraoperative adjuncts, this can provide additional information to the neurosurgeon to facilitate safe and better extent of resection.

References

1. Ophir J, Cespedes I, Ponnekanti H et al (1991) Elastography: a quantitative method for imaging the elasticity of biological tissues. Ultrason Imaging 13(2):111–134
2. Nightingale KR, Palmeri ML, Nightingale RW et al (2001) On the feasibility of remote palpation using acoustic radiation force. J Acoust Soc Am [Internet] 110(1):625
3. Bercoff J, Tanter M, Fink M (2004) Supersonic shear imaging: a new technique for soft tissue elasticity mapping. IEEE Trans Ultrason Ferroelectr Freq Control 51(4):396–409
4. Gebo KA, Herlong HF, Torbenson MS et al (2002) Role of liver biopsy in management of chronic hepatitis C: a systematic review. Hepatology 36(5 (Suppl 1)):S161–S172
5. Sandrin L, Fourquet B, Hasquenoph J-M et al (2003) Transient elastography: a new noninvasive method for assessment of hepatic fibrosis. Ultrasound Med Biol 29(12):1705–1713
6. Cosgrove D, Piscaglia F, Bamber J et al (2013) EFSUMB guidelines and recommendations on the

clinical use of ultrasound elastography. Part 2: clinical applications. Ultraschall Med 34(3):238–253

7. Itoh A, Ueno E, Tohno E et al (2006) Breast disease: clinical application of US elastography for diagnosis. Radiology 239(2):341–350

8. Cho N, Jang M, Lyou CY et al (2012) Distinguishing benign from malignant masses at breast US: combined US elastography and color Doppler US – influence on radiologist accuracy. Radiology 262(1):80–90

9. Berg WA, Cosgrove DO, Doré CJ et al (2012) Shearwave elastography improves the specificity of breast US: the BE1 multinational study of 939 masses. Radiology 262(2):435–449

10. Bojunga J, Herrmann E, Meyer G et al (2010) Realtime elastography for the differentiation of benign and malignant thyroid nodules: a meta-analysis. Thyroid 20(10):1145–1150

11. Veyrieres JB, Albarel F, Lombard JV et al (2012) A threshold value in Shear Wave elastography to rule out malignant thyroid nodules: a reality? Eur J Radiol 81(12):3965–3972

12. Bhatia KSS, Tong CSL, Cho CCM et al (2012) Shear wave elastography of thyroid nodules in routine clinical practice: preliminary observations and utility for detecting malignancy. Eur Radiol 22(11):2397–2406

13. Albert FK, Forsting M, Sartor K et al (1994) Early postoperative magnetic resonance imaging after resection of malignant glioma: objective evaluation of residual tumor and its influence on regrowth and prognosis. Neurosurgery 34(1):45–61

14. Orringer D, Lau D, Khatri S et al (2012) Extent of resection in patients with glioblastoma: limiting factors, perception of resectability, and effect on survival. J Neurosurg 117(5):851–859

15. Golfinos JG, Fitzpatrick BC, Smith LR et al (1995) Clinical use of a frameless stereotactic arm: results of 325 cases. J Neurosurg 83(2):197–205

16. Dorward NL, Alberti O, Velani B et al (1998) Postimaging brain distortion: magnitude, correlates, and impact on neuronavigation. J Neurosurg 88(4):656–662

17. Chandler WF, Rubin JM (1987) The application of ultrasound during brain surgery. World J Surg 11(5):558–569

18. Gronningsaeter A, Kleven A, Ommedal S et al (2000) SonoWand, an ultrasound-based neuronavigation system. Neurosurgery 47(6):1373–1379; discussion 1379–1380

19. Chakraborty A, Bamber JC, Berry G et al (2004) Intra-operative ultrasound elastography and registered MRI of brain tumours: a feasibility study. In: Proc 3rd international conference on the ultrasonic measurement imaging tissue elasticity, 17–20 Oct 2004

20. Chakraborty A, Berry G, Bamber J et al (2006) Intraoperative ultrasound elastography and registered magnetic resonance imaging of brain tumours: a feasibility study. Ultrasound 14(1):43–9

21. Selbekk T, Bang J, Unsgaard G (2005) Strain processing of intraoperative ultrasound images of brain tumours: initial results. Ultrasound Med Biol 31(1):45–51

22. Selbekk T, Brekken R, Solheim O et al (2010) Tissue motion and strain in the human brain assessed by intraoperative ultrasound in glioma patients. Ultrasound Med Biol 36(1):2–10

23. Selbekk T, Brekken R, Indergaard M et al (2012) Comparison of contrast in brightness mode and strain ultrasonography of glial brain tumours. BMC Med Imaging 12(1):11

24. Uff CE (2011) The evaluation of advanced ultrasound elastographic techniques in neurosurgery. Institute of Cancer Research, University of London

25. Uff CE, Garcia L, Fromageau J et al (2009) Real-time ultrasound elastography in neurosurgery. IEEE Int Ultrasound Symp Proc. IEEE, 20-23 September 2009, 467–470

26. Pesavento A, Lorenz A, Siebers S et al (2000) New real-time strain imaging concepts using diagnostic ultrasound. Phys Med Biol 45:1423–1435

27. Scholz M, Noack V, Pechlivanis I et al (2005) Vibrography during tumor neurosurgery. J Ultrasound Med 24(7):985–992

28. Scholz M, Lorenz A, Pesavento A et al (2007) Current status of intraoperative real-time vibrography in neurosurgery. Ultraschall Med 28(5):493–497

29. Chakraborty A (2007) The development of intraoperative ultrasound elasticity imaging techniques to assist during brain tumour resection. PhD thesis, Academic Department of Clinical Neuroscience, University of London

30. Chakraborty A, Bamber JC, Dorward NL (2012) Slip elastography: a novel method for visualising and characterizing adherence between two surfaces in contact. Ultrasonics 52(3):364–376

31. Chan HW, Chakraborty A, Dorward NL et al (2012) Shear wave elastography of pediatric epileptogenic tumors: preliminary results. In: Eleventh international tissue elasticity conference, Deauville, 2–5 Oct 2012, p 113

32. Chan HW, Uff C, Chakraborty A et al (2013) Visualising epileptogenic zones in children with intraoperative shear wave elastography. In: Fifteenth world federation of neurosurgical societies' world congress of neurological surgery, Seoul, 8–13 Sept 2013

33. Chan HW, Uff C, Chakraborty A et al (2014) Detecting MRI-negative epileptogenic lesions with intra-operative shear wave elastography. In: Thirteenth international tissue elasticity conference, Utah, 7–10 Sept 2014, p 61

34. Chan HW, Pressler R, Uff C et al (2014) A novel technique of detecting MRI-negative lesion in focal symptomatic epilepsy: intraoperative ShearWave Elastography. Epilepsia 55(4):e30–e33

35. Chan HW. Optimising the use and assessing the value of intraoperative shear wave elastography in neurosurgery. PhD thesis, Institute of Neurology, University College London, London. (Awaiting submission)

Erratum to: Contrast-Enhanced Ultrasound (CEUS) in Neurosurgery

Francesco Prada, Massimiliano Del Bene, and Francesco DiMeco

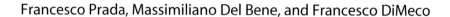

Erratum to:
Chapter 13 in F. Prada et al. (eds.), Intraoperative Ultrasound (IOUS) in Neurosurgery:
From Standard B-mode to Elastosonography, DOI 10.1007/978-3-319-25268-1_13

It was noted that the order of the authors was represented incorrectly. The correct order of the authors should read as follows:

Francesco Prada, Massimiliano Del Bene, and Francesco DiMeco

Also, the header data for this chapter was changed from M. Del Bene et al. to F. Prada et al.

The online version of the updated chapter can be found under
DOI 10.1007/978-3-319-25268-1_13

F. Prada • M. Del Bene, MD (✉)
Department of Neurosurgery, Fondazione IRCCS
Istituto Neurologico C. Besta,
via Celoria 11, Milan 20133, Italy
e-mail: macs.delbene@gmail.com

F. DiMeco
Department of Neurosurgery, Fondazione IRCCS
Istituto Neurologico C. Besta,
via Celoria 11, Milan 20133, Italy

Department of Neurosurgery,
Johns Hopkins Medical School, Baltimore, MD, USA

© Springer International Publishing Switzerland 2016
F. Prada et al. (eds.), *Intraoperative Ultrasound (IOUS) in Neurosurgery:*
From Standard B-mode to Elastosonography, DOI 10.1007/978-3-319-25268-1_15